theclinics.com

FOOT AND ANKLE CLINICS

Tendon Injury and Repair

GUEST EDITOR

Terry S. Saxby, FRACS (Orth)

CONSULTING EDITOR

Mark S. Myerson, MD

December 2007 • Volume 12 • Number 4

SAUNDERS

An Imprint of Elsevier, Inc.

PHILADELPHIA LONDON TORONTO MONTREAL SYDNEY TOKYO

MT

W.B. SAUNDERS COMPANY
A Division of Elsevier Inc.

1600 John F. Kennedy Blvd., Suite 1800, Philadelphia, PA 19103-2899

http://www.theclinics.com

FOOT AND ANKLE CLINICS
December 2007
Editor: Debora Dellapena

Volume 12, Number 4
ISSN 1083-7515
ISBN 1-4160-5071-X
978-1-4160-5071-1

Reprints. For copies of 100 or more of articles in this publication, please contact the Commercial Reprints Department, Elsevier Inc., 360 Park Avenue South, New York, New York 10010-1710. Tel.: (212) 633-3813; Fax: (212) 462-1935, e-mail: reprints@elsevier.com

Foot and Ankle Clinics (ISSN 1083-7515) is published quarterly by Elsevier, Inc., 360 Park Avenue South, New York, NY 10010-1710. Months of issue are March, June, September, and December. Business and Editorial Offices: 1600 John F. Kennedy Blvd., Suite 1800, Philadelphia, PA 19103-2899. Customer Service Office: 6277 Sea Harbor Drive, Orlando, FL 32887-4800. Periodicals postage paid at New York, NY, and additional mailing offices. Subscription prices are $345.00 per year Institutional, $297.00 per year Institutional USA, $345.00 per year Institutional Canada, $283.00 per year Personal, $209.00 per year Personal USA, $234.00 per year Personal Canada, $136.00 per year Personal student, $105.00 per year Personal student USA, $136.00 per year Personal student Canada. To receive student/resident rate, orders must be accompanied by name of affiliated institution, date of term, and the *signature* of program/residency coordinator on institution letterhead. Orders will be billed at individual rate until proof of status is received. Foreign air speed delivery is included in all *Clinics* subscription prices. All prices are subject to change without notice. POSTMASTER: Send address changes to *Foot and Ankle Clinics*, Elsevier Periodicals Customer Service, 6277 Sea Harbor Drive, Orlando, FL 32887-4800. **Customer Service: 1-800-654-2452 (US). From outside of the US, call 1-407-345-1000.**

Printed in the United States of America.

4/2/08

CONSULTING EDITOR

MARK S. MYERSON, MD, Director, The Institute for Foot and Ankle Reconstruction, Mercy Medical Center, Baltimore, Maryland

GUEST EDITOR

TERRY S. SAXBY, MB, BS, FRACS (Orth), Orthopedic Surgeon, Brisbane Foot and Ankle Centre, Brisbane Private Hospital, Brisbane, Australia

CONTRIBUTORS

ADAM AJIS, MRCS, Department of Trauma and Orthopaedic Surgery, Keele University School of Medicine, Staffs, England

J.D.F. CALDER, MD, FRCS (Tr&Orth), FFSEM (UK), Consultant Orthopaedic Surgeon, North Hampshire Hospital, Basingstoke; Clinical Senior Lecturer, Imperial College, London, United Kingdom

MARK DAVIES, FRCS (Tr&Orth), London Foot and Ankle Centre, Hospital of St. John and St. Elizabeth, London, United Kingdom

VINCENZO DENARO, MD, Department of Orthopaedic and Trauma Surgery, Campus Biomedico University, Rome, Italy

R.R. ELLIOT, MA, MRCS, Specialist Registrar, Trauma and Orthopaedics, Royal Bournemouth Hospital, Bournemouth, United Kingdom

CESAR GAMBA, MD, Attending Orthopaedic Surgeon, The Institute for Foot and Ankle Reconstruction, Mercy Medical Center, Baltimore, Maryland

MICHAEL S. HENNESSY, BSc, FRCSEd (Tr&Orth), Consultant Orthopaedic Surgeon, Wirral Hospitals NHS Trust, Upton, Wirral, United Kingdom

MATTHEW HOPE, BScMedSci, MBChB, FRCSEd (Tr&Orth), Fellow in Foot and Ankle Surgery, Brisbane Foot and Ankle Centre, Brisbane Private Hospital, Brisbane, Australia; Clinical Lecturer; and Honorary Specialist Registrar in Orthopaedics, University of Aberdeen, Aberdeen, Scotland, United Kingdom

UMILE GIUSEPPE LONGO, MD, Department of Orthopaedic and Trauma Surgery, Campus Biomedico University, Rome, Italy

NICOLA MAFFULLI, MD, MS, PhD, FRCS, Professor, Department of Trauma and Orthopaedic Surgery, Keele University School of Medicine, Staffs, England

ANDREW P. MOLLOY, FRCS (Tr&Orth), Specialist Registrar, Royal Liverpool University Hospital, Liverpool, United Kingdom

MARK S. MYERSON, MD, Director, The Institute for Foot and Ankle Reconstruction, Mercy Medical Center, Baltimore, Maryland

JOHN P. NEGRINE, MB, BS, FRACS, Foot and Ankle Surgeon, Orthosports, Sydney, Australia

PETER ROSENFELD, MB, BS, FRCS (Tr&Orth), Consultant Foot and Ankle Surgeon, St Mary's Hospital, London, England

TERRY S. SAXBY, MB, BS, FRACS (Orth), Orthopedic Surgeon, Brisbane Foot and Ankle Centre, Brisbane Private Hospital, Brisbane, Australia

H.K. SLATER, MB, BS, FRACS, FAOrthA, Consultant Orthopaedic Surgeon, North Sydney Orthopaedic and Sports Medicine Centre, Sydney, Australia

MATTHEW SOLAN, FRCS (Tr&Orth), London Foot and Ankle Centre, Hospital of St. John and St. Elizabeth, London; Department of Orthopaedic Surgery, Royal Surrey County Hospital; and Surrey Foot and Ankle Clinic, Guildford Nuffield Hospital, Stirling Road, Guildford, Surrey, United Kingdom

NATALIE SQUIRES, MD, InMotion Clinic, Longview, Washington

SIMON W. STURDEE, FRCS (Tr&Orth), Foot and Ankle Fellow, Wirral Hospitals NHS Trust, Upton, Wirral, United Kingdom

CONTENTS

FORTHCOMING ISSUES

March 2008

External Fixation for Lower Limb Salvage
Paul Cooper, MD, *Guest Editor*

June 2008

The Cavovarus Foot
John S. Early, MD, *Guest Editor*

RECENT ISSUES

September 2007

Rheumatoid Arthritis in Foot and Ankle Surgery
Clifford L. Jeng, MD, *Guest Editor*

June 2007

Advances in Posterior Tibial Tendon Insufficiency
Christopher P. Chiodo, MD, *Guest Editor*

March 2007

Complex Salvage of Ankle and Hindfoot Deformity
John G. Anderson, MD and Donald R. Bohay, MD, *Guest Editors*

ELSEVIER
SAUNDERS

Foot Ankle Clin N Am
12 (2007) ix–x

FOOT AND
ANKLE CLINICS

Foreword

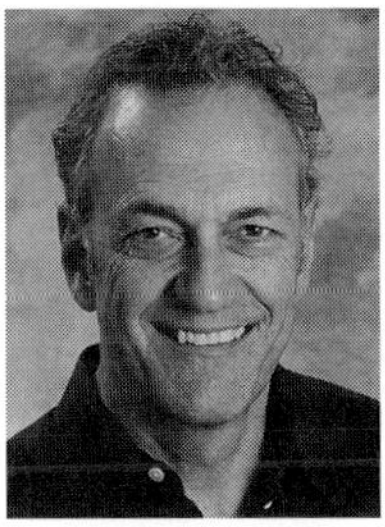

Mark S. Myerson, MD
Consulting Editor

It is interesting how certain procedures do not change much over time. Tendon repair has been performed successfully for decades, and while the suture technique may have evolved regardless of the tendon treated, the principles of treatment remain similar.

It would seem today that the age-old repeated question of management of an acute rupture of the *Achilles tendon* has been resolved, and there are very few proponents worldwide who advocate a closed method of treatment. Accurate restoration of function depends on anatomic restoration of tendon ends and a functional method of rehabilitation, both of which are not possible with closed method of repair. One significant change in my approach to treatment has been with the position of immobilization of the foot during and following repair. Surgeons used to place the sutures in such a manner that the foot matched the opposite limb with respect to dynamic plantar flexion at rest. This ensured that the repair was done in the correct position, which seemed appropriate. However, over time I have realized that some stretching out of this repair always occurs, leading to weakness in push off strength. There is, of course, a physiologic basis for this elongation, but it highlights the importance of the tension applied to the repair. Dynamic rehabilitation with resumption of early protected weight bearing following tendon repair is also important. There are numerous biologic and clinical studies that demonstrate the advantages of early resumption of stress and load on the repaired tendon. While this is most important following repair of the Achilles tendon rupture, the position of the foot in the boot

doi:10.1016/j.fcl.2007.08.001

(clearly not a cast) is also important. It does no good to position the foot in plantar flexion if the boot is also in plantar flexion. This causes an extension stress on the knee, and it will create too much load on the repaired tendon. Instead, use a boot that is locked in neutral, but position the foot in varying degrees of equinus using soft pads inside the boot to vary the load on the tendon.

The current management of ruptures of the *peroneal tendons* has evolved over the past decade. The consequences of a delayed diagnosis of a peroneal tendon rupture, whether the longus, brevis, or both tendons are now recognized, and the biomechanical consequences of chronic rupture are better understood. In particular, rupture of both peroneal tendons ultimately produces heel varus and ankle instability, and a careful intraoperative plan must be followed to restore function. This plan includes an osteotomy of the calcaneus, ankle ligament reconstruction (either with a remnant of the peroneal tendon or an allograft reconstruction), and then restoration of eversion strength either with a transfer of the flexor digitorum longus or an allograft tendon hooked into the remaining peroneal tendon proximally.

Finally, *fixation of tendon* to bone has evolved as well. Suture to bone is not ideal since the healing potential and stability of this type of repair will fail. It is also difficult to correctly tension the tendon when applying a suture to the bone at the same time. A preferable method of attachment is through a tunnel drilled or trephined into a bone and the tendon pulled out the opposite end of the bone so that appropriate tension can be applied. In the past surgeons used the trephine of bone inserted back into the tunnel to hold the tendon, but now this is supplemented either by insertion of a bio-resorbable screw or a bone suture anchor into the tunnel.

Mark S. Myerson, MD
Director
The Institute for Foot and Ankle Reconstruction
Mercy Medical Center
301 St Paul Place
Baltimore, MD 21202, USA

E-mail address: mark4feet@aol.com

ELSEVIER
SAUNDERS

Foot Ankle Clin N Am
12 (2007) xi

FOOT AND
ANKLE CLINICS

Preface

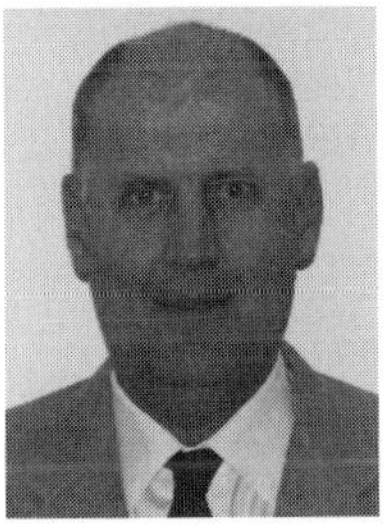

Terry S. Saxby, MB, BS, FRACS (Orth)
Guest Editor

Tendon problems are a common cause of foot and ankle pathology. In the past decade there have been significant advances in the management of these problems. This has been achieved not only by an improvement of surgical techniques, but also through a better understanding of tendon injury and healing.

This issue reviews the recent advances in the diagnosis and treatment of common tendon problems, beginning with a review of tendon healing.

I believe that this issue will provide the reader with an excellent review of all that is new on this topic. The aim is to provide the reader with an up-to-date, concise, but comprehensive review on the topic written by a group of experts. I believe that this goal has been achieved in this issue.

Terry S. Saxby, MB, BS, FRACS (Orth)
Brisbane Foot and Ankle Centre
Brisbane Private Hospital
259 Wickham Terrace
Brisbane, 4069 Australia

E-mail address: forefoot@bigpond.com

doi:10.1016/j.fcl.2007.08.003

ELSEVIER
SAUNDERS

Foot Ankle Clin N Am
12 (2007) 553–567

FOOT AND
ANKLE CLINICS

Tendon Healing

Matthew Hope, BScMedSci, MBChB, FRCSEd (Tr&Orth)[a,b,*], Terry S. Saxby, MB, BS, FRACS (Orth)[a]

[a]*Brisbane Foot and Ankle Centre, Brisbane Private Hospital, 259 Wickham Terrace, Brisbane, 4069, Australia*

[b]*University of Aberdeen, Polwarth Building, Foresterhill, Aberdeen AB25 2ZD, Scotland, UK*

An understanding of the processes of tendon healing and tendon-to-bone healing is important for the intraoperative and postoperative management of patients with tendon ruptures or of patients requiring tendon transfers in foot and ankle surgery. Knowledge of the normal process allows clinicians to develop strategies when normal healing fails. This article reviews the important work behind the identification of the normal phases and control of tendon healing. It outlines the failed response in tendinopathy and describes tendon-to-bone healing in view of its importance in foot and ankle surgery.

Intrinsic and extrinsic tendon healing

Significant advances have been made in the understanding of tendon healing over the last 25 years. Before the early 1970s, it was believed that "the entire flexor tendon callus" originated from the synovial sheath and that the tendon stump was inactive [1]. As a result of this "extrinsic" healing process, where vessels and fibroblasts were believed to migrate from the sheath, the formation of adhesions was felt to be inevitable. The strength of a tendon repair was thought to be insufficient to allow mobilization before 3 weeks. At the time, it was believed that a suture strong enough to allow mobilization would create further problems in the form of connective tissue reaction or even tendon necrosis. Controversy existed as to the role of the epitenon in tendon healing. All tendon healing was initially

* Corresponding author. University of Aberdeen, Polwarth Building, Foresterhill, Aberdeen AB25 2ZD, Scotland, UK.

E-mail address: m.j.hope@abdn.ac.uk (M. Hope).

1083-7515/07/$ - see front matter
doi:10.1016/j.fcl.2007.07.003

believed to be due to fibroblast ingrowth from the tendon sheath. This belief was a result of the observation, on longitudinal sections, of fibroblast growth arising from the synovial sheath without evidence of cellular proliferation occurring at the epitenon [2]. In contrast, early evidence from a healing tendon repair within an isolating tube indicated thickened layers of fibroblasts, demonstrating that a proliferative response may have taken place within the epitenon [1].

Work published in the 1980s confirmed that in contrast to "extrinsic" tendon healing, tendons could undergo primary healing when isolated from the tendon sheath [3,4]. An in vitro experiment using electron microscopy examined divided rabbit flexor tendons in a culture medium. This showed that epitenon cells have the ability to phagocytose collagen and migrate into the laceration site [5]. In addition to migration, cellular proliferation and collagen synthesis was demonstrated in vivo by the transplantation of a divided rabbit flexor tendon to a subcutaneous pocket on the back of each animal [6]. The tendon was placed in a silicone tube and the ends were covered with a semipermeable membrane with a pore size of less than 1 μm in diameter to prevent any cellular infiltration. A proliferation of epitenon cells and the production of collagen were seen at the tendon laceration site within the tube. The observation of tendon healing in the absence of a synovial sheath or outside cellular migration provided further evidence for the intrinsic healing capacity of flexor tendons.

By excluding the synovium, the above experiments confirmed that a tendon had the potential to heal primarily. Because tendon healing within the synovial sheath was associated with adhesion formation, it was not until the effect of mobilization on the cellular changes had been demonstrated that the postoperative management of tendon repairs changed. In a canine study following flexor tendon repair, the animals that had controlled passive mobilization developed a smooth gliding surface of epitenon cells by 10 days. This was in contrast to the immobilized animals, where it was observed that there had been fibroblast ingrowth from the synovium with the resultant formation of adhesions [7]. These adhesions had not resolved at the end of the experiment at 42 days. The cellular changes at the tendon repair surface indicated more active protein synthesis at 21 and 42 days in the animals where controlled passive motion had been used, in comparison to a predominance of collagen resorption in the immobilized tendons. The identification of some of the cellular changes occurring during intrinsic tendon healing explains the observation that controlled mobilization increases the strength and excursion of repaired flexor tendons [8,9].

As a result of this work, the aim of surgical repair of divided healthy tendons contained in a synovial sheath has been to favor intrinsic healing by a repair that is strong enough and smooth enough to allow early mobilization. Despite careful technique and postoperative guidance, complications still occur. The most common complication is the formation of adhesions [10]. The healing process is a balance between the intrinsic and extrinsic healing processes. The mechanism for achieving this balance may lie in the differential ability of the cells to respond to local factors. Collagen production occurs at three sites—the endotenon, the epitenon, and the tendon sheath. Each cell line responds differently to the amount of collagen produced in response to increasing lactate concentration, which is produced during the inflammatory process. The tendon sheath cells increase collagen I production by 70% from baseline compared with only 15% and 12% by the epitenon and endotenon respectively [11]. External influences, such as the extent of the injury, amount of surgical trauma, and the ability to obtain mobilization in the postoperative period, may affect the concentration and distribution of local factors and therefore the magnitude and location of collagen synthesis and resultant adhesion formation.

The phases of tendon healing

Following an acute injury, an inflammatory response initiates the healing process, which passes through a number of overlapping cellular phases. These phases have been subdivided for ease of description. The duration of each phase can vary according to the site, type of injury, and associated drug treatment [12]. The phases are commonly described as the inflammatory, proliferative, and remodelling phases.

The inflammatory phase

The inflammatory phase occurs almost immediately after tendon injury and begins with hematoma formation as a result of vessel damage at the site of injury. The aggregation of platelets causes the release of pro-inflammatory mediators, exposure of adhesion molecules, and recruitment of leukocytes. Phagocytic neutrophils are the first cells to be recruited to the injury site, where they themselves can release cytokines that attract macrophages. The concentration of neutrophils declines after the first 24 hours and thereafter the macrophage is the predominant cell line until the end of the inflammatory phase [13]. Activated macrophages can release growth factors known to induce extracellular matrix formation and can stimulate fibroblasts to proliferate [14]. During this phase, macrophage phagocytosis occurs to remove necrotic tissue and to break down the blood clot. Angiogenesis is then stimulated by the release of promoting factors for the later formation of capillary networks. The importance of reestablishing a capillary network for the delivery of oxygen to the repair site is illustrated by the fact that collagen synthesis is a highly oxygen-dependent process [15].

Proliferative phase

The initial inflammatory phase merges with the following proliferative phase. Animal models of flexor tendon repair reveal that epitenon cells proliferate 3 days after the repair and form a thickened layer 2 to 5 cells deep [16]. The earliest proliferation is seen at the cut ends of the tendon and suture tracks [17]. The epitenon cells (as fibroblasts) lie longitudinally and migrate to the superficial areas of the repair surface associated with an increase in fibronectin activity. The activity of fibronectin, a cellular chemotactic substance and cell attachment molecule, isolates to the epitenon and repair site and does not increase on the endotenon cells [16]. The proliferation of fibroblasts continues so that the epitenon layer reaches 15 to 20 cells thick. The thickening response of the epitenon is very localized. Five millimeters proximally or distally from the repair site, the epitenon has thinned to only 5 or 10 cells thick [16]. At 7 days following flexor tendon repair, evidence of neovascularization has been seen with the formation of vascular channels extending into the repair site [18]. A moderate increase in cellularity occurs in the endotenon, but the predominant proliferative response is in the epitenon and at the superficial areas of the repair site. DNA synthesis, reflecting cell proliferation, has been measured using radiolabelled thymidine. DNA synthesis is greatest at 10 days after repair of the tendon. The levels from the tendon, however, are a third of those found in the surrounding tendon sheath [19].

The study by Wiig and colleagues [19] demonstrated that the time for maximal collagen synthesis after tendon repair was at 10 days. Oshiro and colleagues [18] observed that, between 14 and 21 days following repair, collagen bundles degraded on a massive scale and this degradation was accompanied by the longitudinal arrangement of cells at the epitenon. In the region adjacent to the tendon surface, newly synthesized fine collagen fibers were seen to cross the repair site. Earlier studies indicated that type I collagen is expressed initially by the epitenon cells and later by the teknocytes [17]. More recently, the use of the reverse transcription polymerase chain reaction has allowed the identification of messenger RNA for collagen subtypes from animal models of tendon repair [18,20,21]. These models have indicated that gene expression for type I collagen in the healing tendon initially decreases, but gradually returns to normal after 3 weeks. The production of type III (and also types V and XII) remained persistently elevated during the healing process. Proteoglcan and noncollagenous proteins are also synthesized at increased rates 10 days after the tendon repair [19]. The productions of collagens, noncollagenous proteins, and proteoglycan in the extracellular matrix coincide with the increase in the strength of the healing tendon [22]. The greatest cellular proliferation and vascularity of the repair site is found at 28 days after tendon repair [18]. During the first few weeks following repair, the strength of the tendon increases significantly. In a rabbit model, the mean load to failure of the repair at 4 weeks increased by a factor of eight from 20 N to 166 N. In addition, it was found that during this period there was no significant difference in the strength between the repairs using 4-0 polydioxanone or 4-0 prolene sutures [23].

Remodelling phase

The remodelling of tendon tissue is a slow, non-reactive process that is easily overlooked. Its importance lies in the fact that the end result is a functional scar, which has properties that resemble the original tissue. The remodelling period is believed to begin at the peak of the proliferative phase, but may start as early as 1 or 2 weeks after injury. The remodelling phase is characterized by progressive alignment and organization of the collagen fibrils into bundles. The collagen fibrils, predominantly of type III collagen, are resorbed because of the action of collagenases and are replaced with type I collagen, which has more cross-links and greater tensile strength. The bundles are oriented in the longitudinal axis of the tendon. During this phase, a change from a cellular to a predominantly fibrous tissue takes place in the first few weeks. The large round cells that are initially interposed between the fibrils become increasingly elongated until they resemble mature teknocytes [18]. The final phase of remodelling is maturation. This is a long process and terminates with a gradual decline in tendon vascularity and tenocyte metabolism and a steady increase in collagen bundle thickness. The biomechanical properties of a repaired tendon may continue to improve up to a year after the injury. The tensile strength of the repaired tendon does not match that of the preinjury tendon. In an ovine model, Achilles tendons were allowed to heal spontaneously after transection. The force required to cause rupture at 1 year was only 57% of the force needed to rupture a normal tendon [24].

Tendon healing control

Many physical factors and chemical mediators initiate, sustain, and eventually terminate the complex process of tendon healing. The inflammatory process is initiated by the insult to the tissue, the nature of which is usually mechanical, but may include chemical or thermal injury. The initial insult results in the activation of interlinked vascular and cellular cascades. The immediate vasoconstriction is followed by a period of vasodilatation that persists through the inflammatory phase. The vasodilation is maintained by both chemical means (histamine, prostaglandins, and complement cascade components C3 and C5) and additional influence from the autonomic nervous system. Increased vasopermeability causes the formation of tissue edema and allows exudate release for the formation of a fibrin clot. The increase in permeability is mediated by the release of histamine, serotonin, bradykinin, and prostaglandins.

The cellular response is controlled by factors that can induce chemotaxis and factors that regulate cellular proliferation and protein turnover. Many chemical mediators have been identified as having a chemotactic role. One such mediator is platelet-derived growth factor (PDGF), which is released from damaged platelets. PDGF has been shown to up-regulate the messenger RNA that codes for a subunit of intergrin, the cellular binding protein [25]. Components of the complement cascade, leukotrienes (from macrophages and mast cells) and lymphokines (from polymorphs) have also been identified as playing a part in chemotaxis [26].

The proliferative phase is characterized by cellular changes that result in fibroplasia and angiogenesis. The fibroplasia is partly controlled by growth factors and partly influenced by oxygen and lactic acid levels. The growth factors, such as insulin-like growth factor-1 (IGF-1) and transforming growth factor–β (TGF-β), are released during the inflammatory phase from macrophages but act during the proliferative phase (Table 1). Oxygen and lactate contribute to the control of healing and collagen synthesis. The rate of collagen synthesis decreases in the presence of hypoxia [15]. The exact mechanism by which oxygen and lactate act on collagen synthesis is unclear, but it may occur via effects on growth factors. The levels of lactate and oxygen are critical to collagen synthesis. In wound healing, elevated lactate levels cause a rise in interleukin-1β and growth factors (vascular endothelial growth factor (VEGF) and TGF-β). In contrast, a rise in the level of IGF-1 is associated with an increase in the deposition of collagen [27]. The process of angiogenesis is similarly regulated by growth factors (PDGF, VEGR, and basic fibroblast growth factor). It has been demonstrated that the concentration of messenger RNA for VEGF in cells at the injury site is six times that found in normal epitenon [28]. Angiogenesis can also be stimulated by low tissue oxygen concentration because VEGF levels are known to increase in the presence of hypoxia [29].

Table 1
Roles of growth factors in tendon and ligament healing

Growth factor	Phase	Effect
PDGF	Immediately postinjury, proliferation, and remodelling	Helps stimulate production of other growth factors and has role in tissue remodelling
TGF-β	Inflammatory	Regulates cellular migration and proliferation, proteinase expression, fibronectin binding interactions, termination of cell proliferation, and stimulation of collagen production
IGF-I	Inflammatory, proliferative	Aids fibroblast proliferation and migration; stimulates matrix production
Vascular endothelial growth factor	Postinflammatory, proliferation, and remodeling	Stimulates angiogenesis
Basic fibroblast growth factor	Proliferation and remodeling	Stimulates angiogenesis and regulates cell migration and proliferation

Data from Molloy T, Wang Y, Murrell GAC. The roles of growth factors in tendon and ligament healing. Sports Med 2003;33(5):381–94.

In addition to metabolites, growth factors, and cytokines, enzymes known as metalloproteinases have been identified as important regulators of extracellular matrix remodelling. Metalloproteinases are known to be involved in many physiological remodelling processes, such bone turnover, angiogenesis, menstruation, and wound healing [30]. During tendon healing, the level of metalloproteinases changes [31]. The activity of metalloproteinases is prevented by the action of tissue inhibitors of metalloproteinases (TIMPs) [32]. Tendon remodelling may be regulated by a balance between the actions of the metalloproteinases and the TIMPs. An imbalance in this relationship is associated with disruption of tendon collagen [33]. Other cellular mediators, such as cytokines, growth factors, and interleukins, can enhance the production of either metalloproteinases or TIMPs, thereby affecting the balance of the enzymes and resultant tissue remodelling [34].

Tendon healing in degenerate tendons

The phases of tendon healing that have been described represent the changes after a repair of a previously healthy tendon. These processes would be seen in the foot and ankle following either primary injury and repair or tendon transfer. In the foot and ankle, however, conditions involving the Achilles, tibialis posterior, and peroneal tendons are frequently due to tendinopathy or degenerate tendons [35–37]. Treatment regimens for these conditions involve initial conservative management followed by surgery, if required, to obtain relief of symptoms and tendon healing.

Tendinopathy can be divided into an initial acute phase followed by a protracted chronic stage. The acute phase is characterized by inflammatory cell reaction, circulatory impairment to the tendon, and local edema formation [38,39]. Conservative measures, such as decreasing activity, cold packs, and nonsteroidal anti-inflammatory drugs are used with the intention of controlling the inflammatory process. Evidence suggests that, for many patients, conservative management alleviates symptoms and resolves conditions [40]. However, no one has published direct evidence showing the effect of conservative management on the inflammatory process. In some patients, the symptoms are unresolved after conservative treatment. The reasons for this remain unclear. In an 8-year follow-up study of 83 patients with acute or subacute Achilles tendinopathy, conservative therapy was unsuccessful in 29% of patients [41]. In patients who fail to improve following conservative management, the normal healing response appears to be disordered and does not progress through the normal phases. The chronic stage of tendinopathy is characterized by the absence of inflammatory cells and normal collagen deposition [42,43]. The degenerative changes that have been observed are characterized by an abnormal fiber structure and focal hypercellularity. Vascular proliferation was noted to be a feature in 90% of specimens taken from 163 symptomatic patients. These specimens were noted to have a poor healing response [42].

Surgical procedures for tendinopathy may involve tendon transfers [44], tenolysis, or debridement of the degenerate portions of the tendon with tubularization of the remainder. Clinical success of the latter two types of procedure is well recognized, but the exact nature of the healing process is not clear [45,46]. Most of these procedures involve a period of immobilization, which in itself could have a beneficial effect. Postoperative histological evidence of tendon healing is obviously difficult to obtain and therefore has not been published. A model of an Achilles tendon decompression in rabbits has demonstrated that at 6 weeks following surgery there was no change in collagen makeup from the original but normal tendon in these cases [47]. The most striking feature was a uniform increase in vascularity throughout the entire tendon. It is likely that the generalized increase in vascularity produced by the surgical decompression allows degenerate tendons to heal, although this extrapolation from an animal model with normal tendons can only be made cautiously. In contrast to the new vessel formation associated with the healing process in the animal model, localized neovascularization has been observed by Doppler ultrasound to be associated with symptomatic Achilles tendinopathy [48]. The neovascularization has been seen to diminish, rather than increase, alongside improvement of symptoms and therefore has formed the basis of nonoperative treatment with injections of sclerosant [49]. It is not clear if the decrease in neovascularization is coupled with healing of the tendon or merely associated with an improvement in symptoms.

Tendon-to-bone healing

Tendon transfers are commonly performed in foot and ankle surgery and therefore knowledge of the healing process and the relationship between strength and the time since repair is important for the postoperative management of the patient. There are many methods of fixing tendons to bone. Tunnels can be used to create tendon slings. Alternatively, suture buttons or blind-ending tunnels with interference screws may be used. Most research on tendon fixation to bone arises from work on the attachment of anterior cruciate ligament (ACL) allografts to the tibia and femur.

The specific type of cell that initiates the tendon-to-bone healing is unknown. A flexor tendon used as an ACL graft in a rabbit model indicates that there is an accumulation of macrophages, followed by an invasion and repopulation by macrophages, in the first 10 days following grafting. No proliferation of the intrinsic cells of the tendon was seen [50]. In a canine model where a digital extensor tendon was transplanted into a tibial tunnel, serial histological analysis examined sequential changes between 2 and 26 weeks. A layer of cellular, fibrous tissue was noted to lie between the tendon and the bone along the length of the bone tunnel. This layer progressively matured and reorganized during the healing process. The collagen fibers that attached the tendon to the bone were believed to resemble Sharpey fibers. Radiographs demonstrated remodelling of the trabecular bone that surrounded the tendon [51]. Histological specimens retrieved following ACL reconstructions have revealed that alongside a graft fixed with a biodegradable interference screw, a zone of fibrous cartilage between the tendon graft and the lamellar bone had formed. Collagen fibers were seen at the tendon–bone interface. In patients with distant fixation, and therefore relatively mobile ACL grafts, biopsies resembled granulation tissue without insertion of fibers between the tendon tissue and the bony wall [52]. ACL reconstruction using a semitendinosus graft in a sheep model demonstrated that at 8 weeks perpendicular collagen fibers were present and at 12 weeks these were circumferential. By 24 weeks the bone tunnel was well defined and little further change had occurred by 52 weeks. Up to 12 weeks, the pull-out strength was 17% that of controls. The strength as compared with that of the controls had increased at 24 and 52 weeks to 28% and 40% respectively. After 12 weeks, the failure occurred by graft rupture rather than pullout of the tendon from the tunnel [53].

Although the phases of tendon-to-bone healing have not been established in the same detail as in tendon healing after direct repair, a number of factors are known to influence tendon-to-bone healing. The movement between the tendon graft and bone is greatest at the aperture of the bone tunnel. Rodeo and colleagues [54] showed that the rate of healing is proportional to the distance from the aperture. This investigation, coupled with the histology seen in the ACL retrieval specimens, suggests that significant movement of the tendon within the tunnel has an adverse effect on tendon–bone healing. Nicotine has also been shown to delay tendon healing to bone. In a rat model of rotator cuff attachment, the inflammatory process was prolonged, cellular proliferation was reduced, and the collagen expression was decreased in the presence of nicotine administered subcutaneously [55]. In a similar model, traditional nonspecific nonsteroidal anti-inflammatory drugs and cycloxygenase-2–specific nonsteroidal anti-inflammatory drugs significantly delayed collagen organization and maturation in tendon-to-bone healing [56].

To achieve satisfactory healing of the tendon–bone unit, the studies on ACL reconstruction suggest that fixation where tendon movement has been reduced leads to improved healing. To investigate the strength of fixation to small bones, techniques using an interference screw, suture-button fixation, or staple fixation have been compared. The ultimate load to failure was 62.8 ($\pm$ 9.0) N for the interference screws, 13.9 ($\pm$ 3.8) N for the staple fixation, and 23.9 ($\pm$ 2.6) N for the suture-button fixation [57]. In addition to acknowledging the initial superior pull-out strength of the interference screw, knowledge of the final strength of the tendon healing to either cortical or cancellous bone is important. Tendon healing directly to cortical bone or to a cancellous trough has been examined using a model in goats. At 6 and 12 weeks there was no difference in load to failure and stiffness. Collagen continuity between the tendon and bone had been established equally in both groups [58]. Similarly, the pull-out strength of a rabbit Achilles tendon repaired either to the calcaneal cortex or via a bone tunnel was investigated. Following biomechanical testing, there was no difference between the two groups at 1, 2, 4, 6, and 12 weeks. In both groups, Sharpey fibers were seen securing the tendon to the cortical bone. In this study, tendon resorption was seen within the bone tunnel [59]. A long-term histological examination in sheep of patella tendons repaired to bone demonstrated the presence of bridging collagen fibers at 8 weeks and showed that the resultant enthesis was more fibrous than the original. By 104 weeks the collagen fibrils had changed to reflect more the original morphology but the enthesis remained more hypercellular than the original tendon–bone junction [60].

Bioabsorbable interference screw fixation of soft tissue to bone has been used in the shoulder and knee for at least 10 years [61,62]. It has been only more recently that this type of fixation has been used in foot and ankle surgery. Postmortem evidence shows that at 4 months after implantation of a polylactic acid interference screw, there was no evidence of tunnel widening, lytic bone changes, or inflammatory or foreign body reaction [63]. The healing process after bioabsorbable (polylactic acid) or metal interference screw fixation of ACL allografts has been examined in a prospective randomized trial [64]. No statistically significant differences were found in the levels of complement (C5a), complement complex, and interleukin-8 at 6 weeks and 1 year. Four patients of 20 that had bioabsorbable screw fixation had elevated complement in synovial fluid at 6 weeks, but this difference was not significant. Although this study demonstrates that there appears to be no significant difference in the healing process between polylactic bioabsorbable screws and traditional metal screws, concern still exists about the use of polylactic bioabsorbable screws following the publication of reports of sinus track formation due to foreign body tissue reactions [65]. The rate of sterile tissue reaction was reviewed in 2528 patients following the use of either polyglycolic acid or polylactic acid implants. Soft tissue reactions occurred in 5.3% of patients after polyglycolic acid implant use and in only 0.2% after the use of a polylactic acid implant [66]. Polylactic acid implants degrade more slowly than polyglycolic acid implants, which may account for the elevated rate of tissue reactions. In addition to the risks of tissue reaction, the use of bioabsorbable screws in foot and ankle surgery has not obviated the need for implant removal. Three of 15 patients required removal of polylactic acid screws after fixation of a Lisfranc's diastasis [67]. The strength of bioabsorbable screw fixation has been compared with a traditional tendon-to-tendon technique commonly used for tendon transfers in the foot [68]. The load to failure was 279 N in the traditional technique as opposed to 148 N for the bioabsorbable interference screw. Although weaker, the fixation strength of the interference screw is still within the physiological range.

The evidence reviewed suggests that although an interference screw is an adequate method of fixation, a secure fixation of a tendon to cortical or cancellous bone can provide an equally strong tendon–bone unit once healing has taken place. A traditional tendon-to-tendon fixation technique is stronger than a fixation using a bioabsorbable interference screw. The clinician should choose a fixation method that is sufficiently strong to prevent the tendon becoming detached in the postoperative period. Therefore the choice is in part determined by the anatomical location of the transfer and the level of patient compliance.

Future studies

Despite the advances in the understanding of the processes involved in tendon healing, much remains unknown. The development of adhesions continues to be a major limiting factor that prevents the patient from achieving the range of movement established intraoperatively. Recently, an absorbable adhesion barrier, consisting of oxidized regenerated cellulose, has been wrapped around rat Achilles tendons following repair. Macroscopically and histologically the degree of adhesions were reduced [69]. After further in vivo investigation, this product could have useful applications in the foot and ankle. For applications involving the flexor tendons in the hands, refinement of the technique may be required because less space is available in the hand to accommodate the product.

Further understanding of the mediators of tendon healing may allow interventions that can alter or enhance the tendon healing process. Fibroblast growth factor, VEGF, and bone morphogenic proteins have all been identified and their temporal relationship observed in a model of tendon-to-bone healing [70]. Recent work has also demonstrated that tendon-to-bone healing could be enhanced by postoperative treatment with the bisphosphonate alendronate. In canine flexor tendons repaired to their respective insertion sites, the normal bone resorption in the immediate postoperative period was reduced and the pull-out strength at 21 days was 42% of normal in control animals and 78% of normal following systemic alendronate treatment [71]. Tendon repair relies on good surgical technique. However, rupture of the repair is a recognized complication. Failure occurs as a result of gapping at the repair site or by the suture failing at the knot. Suture material coated with bovine collagen type I has been produced specifically for tendon repair. In vitro work has shown that human osteoblasts and tenocytes display significantly greater cellular adhesion and proliferation on coated sutures than do the cells on uncoated sutures [72]. This type of coated suture, once placed, could bind to the tendon tissue and reduce the degree of compression of the tendon created when the transverse limb of the core suture normally slides through the tissue. This could in turn potentially decrease the amount of gapping and enhance the rate of tendon healing.

Continued research and understanding of the tendon healing process and its control will lead to advances in intraoperative techniques and to the possibility of enhancing the rate of healing by promotion of healing regulators.

Summary

This review has outlined the important evidence that established the theories of intrinsic and extrinsic tendon healing. Tendon healing appears to occur by a balance of these processes mediated by multiple local factors. Early mobilization has been shown to decrease adhesion formation and is associated with elevated protein synthesis at the repair site. Studies of the phases of tendon healing indicate that an important step in the remodelling process occurs between 14 and 21 days, when the maximal rate of collagen breakdown is seen. This collagen breakdown is likely to be the cause for early failures of tendon repair that have been insufficiently strong to allow early mobilization.

The studies examining chronic tendinopathy demonstrate an absence of an inflammatory process and normal tendon healing. Although some reports of treatment that reduce the neovascularization associated with tendinopathy demonstrate an improvement in symptoms, the exact mechanism by which this occurs remains unknown. Conservative treatment with surgical debridement in selected cases remains the mainstay of current treatment. The surgical insult of the debridement may have a stimulatory effect that allows the healing to revert to a normal pathway.

Tendon-to-bone healing relies on adequate fixation stronger than the physiological loads applied during the convalescent period. Healing is improved by reducing the movement at the bone–tendon interface. Given these factors, the choice of fixation and site within the bone, whether it is cortical or cancellous, appears to have little significant influence on the outcome with regard to healing. Nicotine and nonsteroidal anti-inflammatory drugs have been shown to reduce the tendon-to-bone healing. Meanwhile, bioabsorbable screws, particularly those with polyglycolic components, remain a concern because of the rate of foreign-body–type reactions and the need for implant removal in some cases.

References

[1] Verdan CE. Half a century of flexor-tendon surgery. Current status and changing philosophies. J Bone Joint Surg Am 1972;54:472–91.

[2] Potenza AD. Tendon healing within the flexor digital sheath in the dog. An experimental study. J Bone Joint Surg Am 1962;44:49–64.

[3] Manske PR, Lesker PA, Gelberman RH, et al. Intrinsic restoration of the flexor tendon surface in nonhuman primate. J Hand Surg [Am] 1985;10:632–7.

[4] Gelberman RH, Manske PR, Akeson WH, et al. Flexor tendon repair. J Orthop Res 1986;4: 119–28.

[5] Manske PR, Gelberman RH, Vande Berg JS, et al. Intrinsic flexor-tendon repair. A morphological study in vitro. J Bone Joint Surg Am 1984;66:385–96.

[6] Lundborg G, Rank F, Heinau B. Intrinsic tendon healing. A new experimental model. Scand J Plast Reconstr Surg Hand Surg 1985;19:113–7.

[7] Gelberman RH, Vande Berg JS, Lundborg GN, et al. Flexor tendon healing and restoration of the gliding surface: an ultrastructural study in dogs. J Bone Joint Surg Am 1983;65:70–80.

[8] Strickland JW, Glogovac SV. Digital function following flexor tendon repair in zone II: a comparison of immobilization and controlled passive motion techniques. J Hand Surg [Am] 1980;5(6):537–43.
[9] Woo SL-Y, Gelberman RH, Cobb NG, et al. The importance of controlled passive mobilization on flexor tendon healing: a biomechanical study. Acta Orthop Scand 1981;52:615–22.
[10] Lilly SI, Messer TM. Complications after treatment of flexor tendon injuries. J Am Acad Orthop Surg 2006;14:387–96.
[11] Klein MB, Pham H, Yalamanchi N, et al. Flexor tendon wound healing in vitro: the effect of lactate tendon cell proliferation and collagen production. J Hand Surg [Am] 2001;26:847–54.
[12] Riley GP, Cox M, Harrell RL, et al. Inhibition of cell proliferation and matrix glycosaminoglycan synthesis by non-steroidal anti-inflammatory drugs in vitro. J Hand Surg [Br] 2001;26:224–8.
[13] Marsolais D, Cote CH, Frenette J. Neutrophils and macrophages accumulate sequentially following Achilles tendon injury. J Orthop Res 2001;19:1203–9.
[14] Fukasawa M, Bryant S, Nakamura RM, et al. Modulation of fibroblast proliferation by postsurgical macrophages. J Surg Res 1987;43:513–20.
[15] Gibson DR, Angeles AP, Hunt TK. Increased oxygen tension on wound metabolism and collagen synthesis. Surg Forum 1997;48:696–9.
[16] Gelberman RH, Steinberg D, Amiel D, et al. Fibroblast chemotaxis after tendon repair. J Hand Surg [Am] 1991;16:686–93.
[17] Garner WL, McDonald JA, Koo M, et al. Identification of the collagen-producing cells in healing flexor tendons. Plast Reconstr Surg 1989;83(5):875–9.
[18] Oshiro W, Lou J, Xing X, et al. Flexor tendon healing in the rat: a histologic and gene expression study. J Hand Surg [Am] 2003;28:814–23.
[19] Wiig M, Abrahamsson SO, Lundborg G. Tendon repair—cellular activities in rabbit deep flexor tendons and surrounding synovial sheaths and the effects of hyaluronan: an experimental study in vivo and in vitro. J Hand Surg [Am] 1997;22:818–25.
[20] Tang JB, Xu Y, Ding F, et al. Expression of genes for collagen production and NF-kappaB gene activation of in vivo healing flexor tendons. J Hand Surg [Am] 2004;29:564–70.
[21] Berglund M, Reno C, Hart DA, et al. Patterns of mRNA expression for matrix molecules and growth factors in flexor tendon injury: differences in the regulation between tendon and tendon sheath. J Hand Surg [Am] 2006;31:1279–87.
[22] McDowell CL, Marqueen TJ, Yager D, et al. Characterisation of the tensile properties and histologic/biochemical changes in normal chicken tendon at the site of suture insertion. J Hand Surg [Am] 2002;27:605–14.
[23] O'Broin ES, Earley MJ, Smyth H, et al. Absorbable sutures in tendon repair. A comparison of PDS with prolene in rabbit tendon repair. J Hand Surg [Br] 1995;20:505–8.
[24] Bruns J, Kampen J, Kahrs J, et al. Achilles tendon rupture: experimental results on spontaneous repair in a sheep-model. Knee Surg Sports Traumatol Arthrosc 2000;8(6):364–9.
[25] Harwood FL, Goomer RS, Gelberman RH, et al. Regulation of alpha(v)beta3 and alpha5-beta 1 integrin receptors by basic fibroblast growth factor and platelet-derived growth factor-BB in intrasynovial flexor tendon cells. Wound Repair Regen 1999;7:381–8.
[26] Derich MP, Forster O, Grunicke H, et al. Inflammation and phagocytosis. J Clin Chem Clin Biochem 1987;25:785–93.
[27] Trabold O, Wagner S, Wicke C, et al. Lactate and oxygen constitute a fundamental regulatory mechanism in wound healing. Wound Repair Regen 2003;11:504–9.
[28] Bidder M, Towler DA, Gelberman RH, et al. Expression of mRNA for vascular endothelial growth factor at the repair site of healing canine flexor tendon. J Orthop Res 2000;18:247–52.
[29] Constant JS, Feng JJ, Zabel DD, et al. Lactate elicits vascular endothelial growth factor from macrophages: a possible alternative to hypoxia. Wound Repair Regen 2000;8:353–60.
[30] Magra M, Maffulli N. Molecular events in tendinopathy: a role for metalloproteases. Foot Ankle Clin 2005;10:267–77.
[31] Birkedal-Hansen H. Proteolytic remodelling of extracellular matrix. Curr Opin Cell Biol 1995;7:728–35.

[32] Gomez DE, Alonso DF, Yoshiji H, et al. Tissue inhibitors of metalloproteinases: structure, regulation and biological functions. Eur J Cell Biol 1997;74:111–22.

[33] Dalton S, Cawston TE, Riley GP, et al. Human shoulder tendon biopsy samples in organ culture produce procollagenase and tissue inhibitor of metalloproteinases. Ann Rheum Dis 1995;54(7):571–7.

[34] Mauviel A. Cytokine regulation of metalloproteinase gene expression. J Cell Biochem 1993; 53:288–95.

[35] Paavola M, Kannus P, Jarvinen TAH, et al. Achille tendinopathy. J Bone Joint Surg Am 2002;84:2062–76.

[36] Goncalves-Neto J, Witzel SS, Teodoro WR, et al. Changes in collagen matrix composition in human posterior tibial tendon dysfunction. Joint Bone Spine 2002;69(2):189–94.

[37] Selmani E, Gjata V, Gjika E. Peroneal tendon disorders. Foot Ankle Int 2006;27(3):221–8.

[38] Puddu G, Ippolito E, Postacchini F. A classification of Achilles tendon disease. Am J Sports Med 1976;4:145–50.

[39] Leach RE, James S, Wasilliewski S. Achilles tendinitis. Am J Sports Med 1981;9:93–8.

[40] Alvarez RG, Marini A, Schmitt C, et al. Stage I and stage II posterior tibial tendon dysfunction treated by a structured non-operative management protocol: an orthosis and exercise program. Foot Ankle Int 2006;27(1):2–8.

[41] Schepsis AA, Wagner C, Leach RE. Surgical management of Achilles tendon overuse injuries. A long term follow-up study. Am J Sports Med 1994;22:611–9.

[42] Astrom M, Rausing A. Chronic Achilles tendinopathy: a survey of surgical and histopathologic findings. Clin Orthop Relat Res 1995;316:151–64.

[43] Maffulli N, Barrass V, Ewen SWB. Light microscopic histology of Achilles tendon ruptures. Am J Sports Med 2001;28:857–63.

[44] Wilcox DK, Bohay DR, Anderson JG. Treatment of chronic tendon disorders with flexor hallucis longus tendon transfer/augmentation. Foot Ankle Int 2000;21(12):1004–10.

[45] Johnston E, Scranton P Jr, Pfeffer GB. Chronic disorders of the Achilles tendon: results of conservative and surgical treatments. Foot Ankle Int 1997;18(9):570–4.

[46] Nelen G, Martens M, Burssens A. Surgical treatment of chronic Achilles tendinitis. Am J Sports Med 1989;17(6):754–9.

[47] Friedrich T, Schmidt W, Junqmichel D, et al. Histopathology in rabbit Achilles tendon after operative tenolysis (longitudinal fiber incisions). Scand J Med Sci Sports 2001;11(1):4–8.

[48] Alfredson H, Ohberg L, Forsgren S. Is vasculo-neural ingrowth the cause of pain in chronic Achilles tendinsis? An investigation using ultrasonagraphy and colour Doppler, immunohistochemistry, and diagnostic injections. Knee Surg Sports Traumatol Arthrosc 2003;11(5): 334–8.

[49] Lind B, Ohberg L, Alfredson H. Sclerosing polidocanol injections in mid-portion Achilles tendinosis: remaining good clinical results and decreased tendon thickness at 2-year follow-up. Knee Surg Sports Traumatol Arthrosc 2006;14(12):1327–32.

[50] Kawamura S, Ying L, Kim HJ, et al. Macrophages accumulate in the early phase of tendon–bone healing. J Orthop Res 2005;23(6):1425–32.

[51] Rodeo SA, Arnoczky SP, Torzilli PA, et al. Tendon-healing in a bone tunnel. A biomechanical and histological study in the dog. J Bone Joint Surg Am 1993;75(12):1795–803.

[52] Nebelung W, Becker R, Urbach D, et al. Histological findings of tendo-bone healing following cruciate ligament reconstruction with hamstring grafts. Arch Orthop Trauma Surg 2003; 123(4):158–63.

[53] Goradia VK, Rochat MC, Grana WA, et al. Tendon-to-bone healing of a semitendinosus autograft used for ACL reconstruction in a sheep model. Am J Knee Surg 2000;13(3):143–51.

[54] Rodeo SA, Kawamura S, Kim HJ, et al. Tendon healing in a bone tunnel differs at the tunnel entrance versus the tunnel exit: an effect of graft-tunnel motion. Am J Sports Med 2006; 34(11):1790–800.

[55] Galatz LM, Silva MJ, Rothermich SY, et al. Nicotine delays tendon-to-bone healing in a rat shoulder model. J Bone Joint Surg Am 2006;88(9):2027–34.

[56] Cohen DB, Kawamura S, Etheshami JR, et al. Indomethacin and colecoxib impair rotator cuff tendon-to-bone healing. Am J Sports Med 2006;34(3):362–9.
[57] Ojuno H, Tanaka J, Fujioka H, et al. Evaluation of an interference screw for tendon reattachment to small bones. J Orthop Trauma 2002;16:418–21.
[58] St Pierre P, Olson EJ, Elliot JJ, et al. Tendon-healing to cortical bone compared with healing to a cancellous trough. A biomechanical and histological evaluation in goats. J Bone Joint Surg Am 1995;77(12):1858–66.
[59] Shaieb MD, Singer DI, Grimes J, et al. Evaluation of tendon-to-bone reattachment: a rabbit model. Am J Orthop 2000;297:537–42.
[60] Newsham-West R, Nicolson H, Walton M, et al. Long-term morphology of a healing bone–tendon interface: a histological observation in the sheep model. J Anat 2007;210(3):318–27.
[61] Barber FA, Elrod BF, McGuire DA, et al. Preliminary results of an absorbable interference screw. Arthroscopy 1995;11(5):537–48.
[62] Shall LM, Cawley PW. Soft tissue reconstruction in the shoulder. Comparison of suture anchors, absorbable staples, and absorbable tacks. Am J Sports Med 1994;22(5):715–8.
[63] McGuire DA, Barber FA, Milchgrub S, et al. A postmortem examination of poly-L lactic acid interference screws 4 months after implantation during anterior cruciate ligament reconstruction. Arthroscopy 2001;17(9):988–92.
[64] Drogset JO, Grontvedt T, Jessen V, et al. Comparison of in vitro and in vivo complement activation by metal and bioabsorbable screws used in anterior cruciate ligament reconstruction. Arthroscopy 2006;22(5):489–96.
[65] Mosier-Laclair S, Pike H, Pomeroy G. Intraosseous bioabsorbable poly-L-lactic acid screw presenting as a late foreign-body reaction: a case report. Foot Ankle Int 2001;22(3):247–51.
[66] Bostman OM, Pihlajamaki HK. Adverse tissue reactions to bioabsorbable fixation devices. Clin Orthop Relat Res 2000;371:216–27.
[67] Saxena A. Bioabsorbable screws for reduction of Lisfranc's diastasis in athletes. J Foot Ankle Surg 2005;44(6):445–9.
[68] Sabonghy EP, Wood RM, Ambrose CG, et al. Tendon transfer fixation: comparing a tendon to tendon technique vs. bioabsorbable interference-fit screw fixation. Foot Ankle Int 2003; 24(3):260–2.
[69] Temiz A, Ozturk C, Bakunov A, et al. A new material for prevention of peritendinous fibrotic adhesions after tendon repair: oxidised regenerated cellulose (Interceed), an absorbable adhesion barrier. Int Orthop 2007;9:Epub ahead of print.
[70] Kohno T, Ishibashi Y, Tsuda E, et al. Immunohistochemical demonstration of growth factors at the tendon–bone interface in anterior cruciate ligament reconstruction using a rabbit model. J Orthop Sci 2007;12(1):67–73.
[71] Thomopoulos S, Matsuzaki H, Zaegel M, et al. Alendronate prevents bone loss and improves tendon-to-bone repair strength in a canine model. J Orthop Res 2007;25(4):473–9.
[72] Mazzocca AD, McCarthy MB, Arciero C, et al. Tendon and bone responses to a collagen-coated suture material. J Shoulder Elbow Surg 2007;18:Epub ahead of print.

ELSEVIER
SAUNDERS

Foot Ankle Clin N Am
12 (2007) 569–572

FOOT AND
ANKLE CLINICS

Tibialis Anterior Rupture: Acute and Chronic

John P. Negrine, MB, BS, FRACS

Orthosports, 160 Belmore Road, Randwick, Sydney, NSW 2031, Australia

The tibialis anterior muscle is the principal dorsiflexor of the ankle. Although overuse tendonitis is not uncommon [1] rupture of the tendon is decidedly rare and few reports in the literature include more than a handful of cases [2].

Anatomy

The tibialis anterior muscle arises from the lateral condyle of the tibia, the proximal half to two thirds of the lateral surface of the tibial shaft, the interosseous membrane, and the deep surface of the fascia cruris. The insertion is to the medial and plantar surfaces of the medial cuneiform and to the base of the first metatarsal.

The vascularity of the tendon has been investigated [3]. There is an avascular zone in the anterior half where the tendon wraps around the superior and inferior retinacula, which serve as fibrous pulleys. A layer of chondroid cells in this region serves to aid the tendon in gliding through the pulleys and is an adaptation to compressive and shearing forces. Not surprisingly, this is the region where most spontaneous ruptures occur.

Although gout, steroid injections, rheumatoid arthritis, and diabetes have been implicated, most patients who rupture have no underlying pathology (Fig. 1).

Clinical presentation

The condition is most common in men between 60 and 80 years of age [1,2,4–6]. A history of minor trauma in plantarflexion is common, where

E-mail address: office@orthosports.com.au

1083-7515/07/$ - see front matter
doi:10.1016/j.fcl.2007.07.004

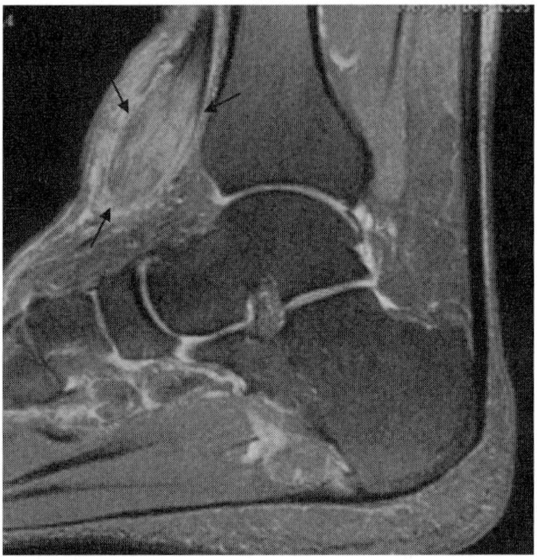

Fig. 1. Tophaceous gout involving the tibialis anterior tendon. Sagittal fat suppressed proton density image demonstrating marked fusiform thickening (*arrows*) of the midfibers of the tibialis anterior tendon and heterogeneous mild signal hyperintensity. (*Courtesy of* J. Linklater, FRANZCR, Sydney, Australia.)

the patient experiences acute pain and feels a "snap." This is invariably accompanied by swelling and then a foot-drop gait with difficulty in walking. The initial symptoms usually resolve in days to weeks, leaving the patient weak but not in any particular pain. Patients may present with a lump at the ankle and not be aware of the weakness, which means that delay in presentation is common.

Physical examination reveals a swelling often localized to the supramalleolar region (where the tendon has retracted). The patient is able to walk on the toes though not on the heels. A high-stepping gait with recruitment of the toe extensors in the swing phase of gait is also observed.

The differential diagnosis of the foot drop observed is a common peroneal nerve lesion or an L5 radiculopathy. Clinically the differentiation of these conditions is usually obvious but investigations such as ultrasound and MRI [7] will readily diagnose the rupture (Fig. 2).

Treatment

The treatment must be tailored to the patient. In the very elderly inactive patient, nonsurgical treatment consisting of an ankle–foot orthosis is suggested. In reality, patients function well though are still weak in dorsiflexion.

In more active patients, a repair results in better function.

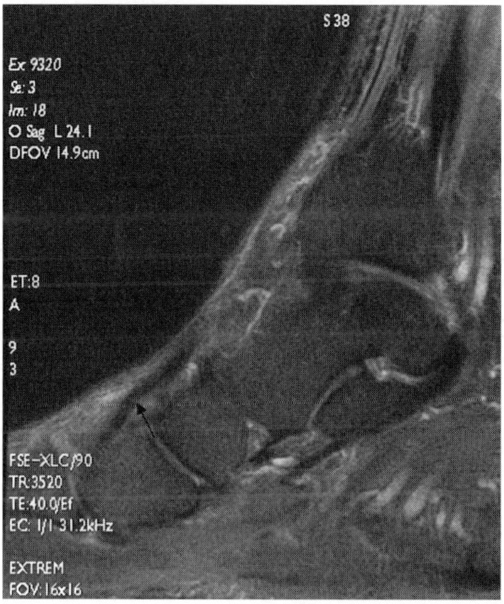

Fig. 2. Distal tibialis anterior tendinosis and partial tear. Sagittal fat suppressed proton density image demonstrating thickening of the distal tibialis anterior tendon and high signal intensity at the deep margin, indicating partial tear (*arrow*). (*Courtesy of* J. Linklater, FRANZCR, Sydney, Australia.)

Acute repair

If diagnosed early (within 1 month) an acute repair may be attempted. Because the tendon is subcutaneous, the surgical approach is longitudinal and medial. The inferior extensor retinaculum is divided and the tendon sheath opened. The distal stump is mobilized and the tendon repaired with a No. 1 nonabsorbable suture. The repair is oversewn with a No. 2-0 absorbable suture. The sheath and extensor retinaculum are then repaired and the patient placed in a non–weight-bearing cast for 6 weeks. At 6 weeks, gentle range-of-motion exercises are commenced. The author prefers a further 3 weeks in a removable boot to protect the repair.

If the distal stump is poor, the tendon may be attached proximally to the medial cuneiform. Numerous techniques are available for the reattachment, including screw and soft tissue washer, pull-out wire, suture anchors, and, recently, an interference fit screw into a drill hole.

Delayed repair

Often patients present late and an acute repair is not possible. The surgery is then directed at either bridging the gap or transferring a tendon to substitute function.

If the remaining tendon is in satisfactory condition, then a slide-lengthening is well described using half the diameter of the tendon. The distal attachment as before is made into bone.

If the tibialis anterior is poor and a slide is not possible, then a repair using extensor hallucis longus (EHL) into the medial cuneiform is performed. The proximal EHL can be sutured to the tibialis anterior if some glide is still present in the tendon. To prevent a "floppy" great toe, the distal EHL is joined to the extensor digitorum longus (EDL) of the second toe. Once again the rehabilitation involves 6 weeks in a cast and 3 in a walking boot.

The alternative transfer described is tibialis posterior through the interosseous membrane.

Summary

Because most patients with this rupture are relatively inactive, nonsurgical treatment is likely to suffice.

In active patients, however, the weakness of dorsiflexion causes significant disability and operative repair should be considered, even in cases of delayed presentation.

References

[1] Negrine J. Disorders of the anterior tibial tendon. Presented at New Zealand Foot and Ankle Society meeting. Lake Taupo, New Zealand, May 16, 2003.
[2] Patten A, Pun WK. Spontaneous rupture of the tibialis anterior tendon: a case report and review of the literature. Foot Ankle Int 2000;21:697–700.
[3] Petersen W, Stein V, Bobka T. Structure of the human tibialis anterior tendon. J Anat 2000; 197(Pt 4):617–25.
[4] Dooley B, Kudelka P, Menelaus M. Subcutaneous rupture of the tendon of tibialis anterior. J Bone Joint Surg Br 1980;62:471–2.
[5] Mankey M. Anterior tibial tendon ruptures. Foot Ankle Clin 1996;1:315–24.
[6] Ouzounian T, Anderson R. Anterior tibial tendon rupture. Foot Ankle Int 1995;16:406–10.
[7] Gallo R, Kolman B, Daffner R, et al. MRI of tibialis anterior tendon rupture. Skeletal Radiol 2004;33:102–6.

ELSEVIER
SAUNDERS

Foot Ankle Clin N Am
12 (2007) 573–582

FOOT AND
ANKLE CLINICS

Percutaneous and Mini-Open Repair of Acute Achilles Tendon Rupture

R.R. Elliot, MA, MRCS[a,*],
J.D.F. Calder, MD, FRCS (Tr&Orth), FFSEM (UK)[b,c]

[a]*Trauma and Orthopaedics, Royal Bournemouth Hospital, Bournemouth BH7 7DW, UK*
[b]*North Hampshire Hospital, Aldermaston Road, Basingstoke RG24 9NA, UK*
[c]*Imperial College, London SW7 2AZ, UK*

The optimal method of treatment and the rehabilitation regime for acute rupture of the Achilles tendon remains controversial [1]. For operative intervention there is further debate regarding which of the described surgical procedures are the most appropriate, most reliable, and safest.

The main concerns regarding conservative treatment has been the incidences of rerupture [2,3], lengthening of the tendon, and poor function [4]. Problems particular to surgery include wound breakdown, infection, scar adhesions, and sural nerve damage. Surgery for the ruptured Achilles tendon has evolved over time in an attempt to improve the functional outcome and reduce the incidence of these complications. There will always be cases for whom conservative therapy is most appropriate and others in whom the percutaneous and mini-open techniques are contraindicated. This article gives an update on percutaneous and mini-open methods for the treatment of acute rupture of the Achilles tendon.

Indications

The techniques described below are recognized treatments for acute rupture of the Achilles tendon. Soon after rupture, the space between the tendon ends fills with hematoma and developing scar tissue, making apposition of the tendon stumps by closed manipulation increasingly difficult. For this reason, delayed presentation is seen as a contraindication to fixation by percutaneous methods. In terms of the timing of surgery, the

* Corresponding author.
E-mail address: rre72@yahoo.co.uk (R.R. Elliot).

doi:10.1016/j.fcl.2007.07.002

indications of the mini-open technique may be extended when compared with pure percutaneous techniques because the rupture site is visualized and interposed hematoma and scar tissue can be removed to allow stump apposition and restoration of appropriate tendon length. Repairs using the Achillon device have been reported up to 3 weeks after injury [5]. Patients with diabetes or vascular disease, smokers, and those taking corticosteroids should be carefully considered on an individual basis. Rupture at the musculotendinous junction and those at the calcaneal insertion are not suitable for repair using percutaneous techniques or the Achillon device. All of the techniques described below can be performed under local anesthetic if necessary.

Techniques: 1977 to present day

Surgical repair of the Achilles tendon was described as early as the tenth century AD [6]. In 1977, Ma and Griffith [7] were the first to describe a technique of percutaneous repair of acute Achilles rupture. It was their intention to reduce the complications associated with open surgery (wound problems and scar adhesions) and lower the rerupture rate reported with conservative treatment [2,3]. Their technique involves making six stab incisions, three on either side of the tendon, and using these incisions to pass a Bunnell suture through the proximal stump and a box suture through the distal stump, thereby affecting a repair (Fig. 1).

In their own series, Ma and Griffith reported only two minor skin complications and no sural nerve damage. A subsequent report on a series of patients treated with this technique showed a worryingly high percentage (13%) of sural nerve damage [8]. The high possibility of sural nerve entrapment using this technique was confirmed in the cadaveric studies of Hockenbury and Johns [9]. They performed percutaneous Achilles tendon repairs on cadaver specimens, using the technique described by Ma and Griffith. In three out of five cases, the sural nerve became trapped by the proximal suture. Anatomical studies have also shown a significant degree of variability in the location of the sural nerve in relation to the Achilles tendon [10,11], further complicating attempts to avoid entrapment. Exposure of the sural nerve during percutaneous repair, by extending the proximal and intermediate stab incisions on the lateral side of the tendon, has been shown to reduce the incidence of nerve injury to zero in a case control study involving 84 patients [12].

Hockenbury and Johns' work also showed that those tendons repaired with an open technique were able to tolerate twice the degree of ankle dorsiflexion before a 10-mm gap appeared in the tendon when compared with those sutured with Ma and Griffith's configuration. In response to this apparent weakness in the Ma and Griffith repair, Cretnik and colleagues [13] devised a modification of the technique that involved starting the suture on

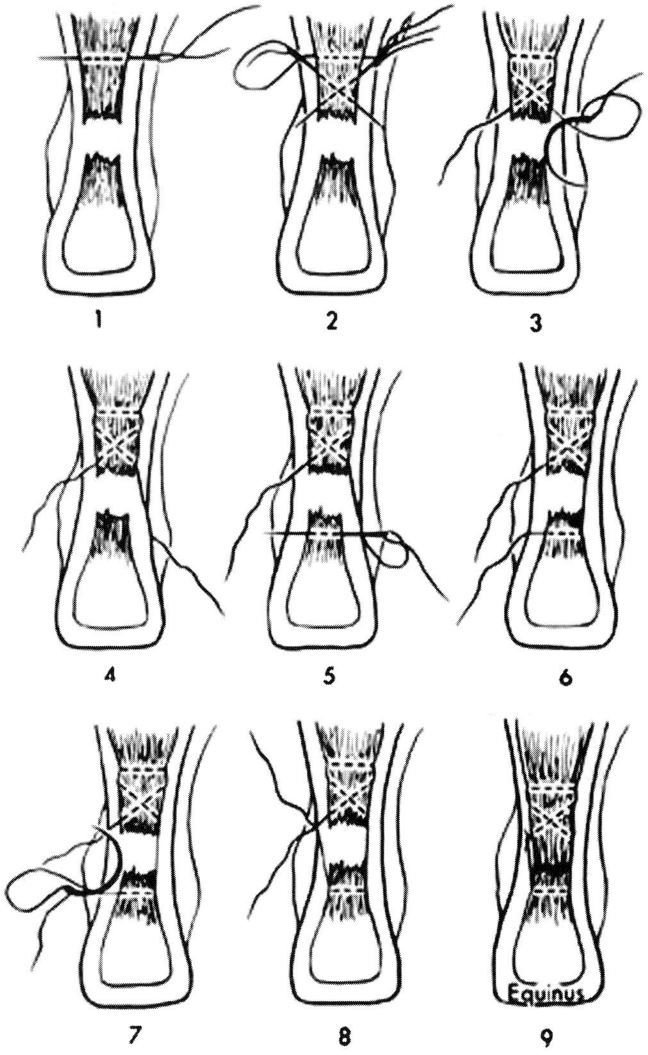

Fig. 1. Ma and Griffith technique for percutaneous repair of acute ruptured Achilles tendon. (*From* Azar FM. Campbell's operative orthopaedics. vol. 3. In: Canale ST, editor. Philadelphia: Mosby; 2003. p. 2463; with permission.)

the medial side at the level of the rupture and included more passes of the suture material through the distal stump. On load testing, this repair significantly improved the gapping resistance at the repair site and the mean load to failure. Cretnik and colleagues have subsequently published a two-cohort study (237 patients) comparing their modified percutaneous technique to a standard open repair [14]. This showed an equivalent functional outcome in both groups but less overall complications in the percutaneous group.

The rate of sural nerve disturbance (4.5% versus 2.8%) and rerupture (3.7% versus 2.8%) were not significantly different between the groups (percutaneous versus open). Lim and colleagues [15] used a similar modification in their randomized controlled study comparing a modified Ma and Griffith's repair to an open repair (Kessler). There were 33 patients per group. No statistically significant difference was shown in the rates of rerupture. There was one sural nerve injury in the percutaneous group (3%), none in the open group. There were significantly more minor complications (infection, adhesion formation, and keloid scaring) in the open group ($P = .01$).

The high percentage of sural nerve injury variably reported amongst patients treated with a Ma and Griffith's repair led Webb and Bannister [16] to develop a new percutaneous technique with the aim of reducing the incidence of this complication. Their technique involves only three skin incisions and these incisions are kept well away from the lateral side of the tendon to protect the sural nerve (Fig. 2).

In their original paper, Webb and Bannister describe a series of 27 patients treated with this method and reported no sural nerve injuries. A retrospective study of 57 patients that compared Webb and Bannister's

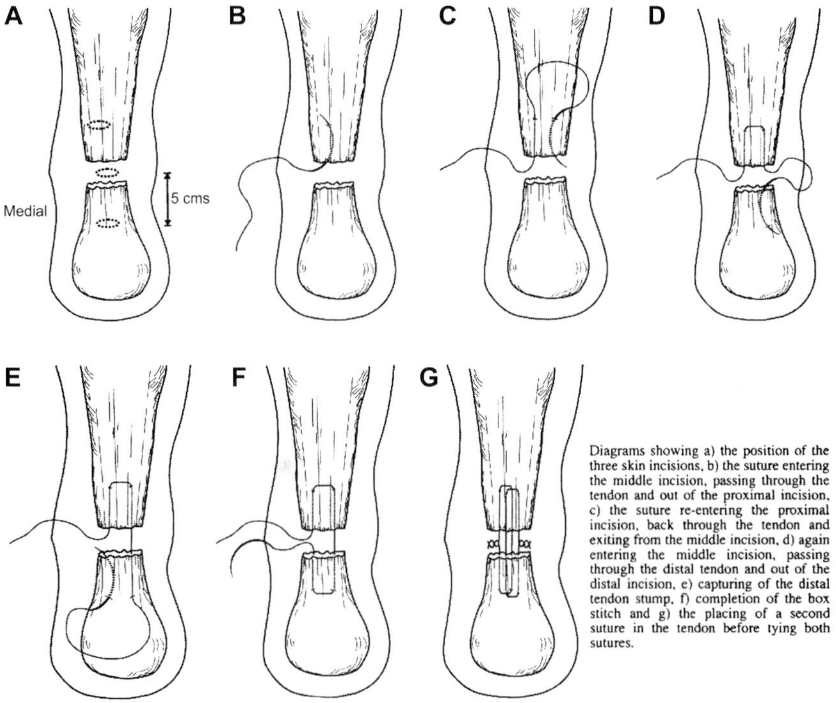

A
B
C
D
Medial
5 cms
E
F
G
Diagrams showing a) the position of the three skin incisions, b) the suture entering the middle incision, passing through the tendon and out of the proximal incision, c) the suture re-entering the proximal incision, back through the tendon and exiting from the middle incision, d) again entering the middle incision, passing through the distal tendon and out of the distal incision, e) capturing of the distal tendon stump, f) completion of the box stitch and g) the placing of a second suture in the tendon before tying both sutures.

Fig. 2. (*A–G*) Webb and Bannister technique. (*From* Webb JM, Bannister GC. Percutaneous repair of the ruptured tendo Achillis. J Bone Joint Surg Br 1999;81(5):878; with permission.)

technique with an open repair showed that the functional results of the Webb–Bannister technique were comparable to those associated with an open repair and there were fewer wound complications [17].

Delponte and colleagues [18] also described a modified percutaneous technique using a harpoon device (Fig. 3). A case series of 124 patients published by Maes and colleagues [19] and using Delponte's Tenolig device (Fournitures Hospitalieres Industrie, Quimper, France) in treating acute Achilles tendon rupture, revealed significant complications, including suture and device failure and a high rate of rerupture (10%) and sural nerve entrapment (5.2%).

Gorschewsky and colleagues [20] modified the "harpoon tenorrhaphy" technique in two ways: (1) They used a small open incision at the rupture site, which they identified using ultrasound, and, (2) after passage of the wires, they used a fibrin sealant to augment the repair. They report more favorable outcomes in their 64 patients with all patients returning to sport after an average 5.5 months, no sural nerve injuries, and only one rerupture due to a further injury.

Several other investigators have recognized that one of the major limitations of the percutaneous technique is an inability to adequately see the rupture site, to clear out hematoma and interposed tissue, and to visualize tendon stump apposition [21–23]. The cadaveric work of Hockenbury and

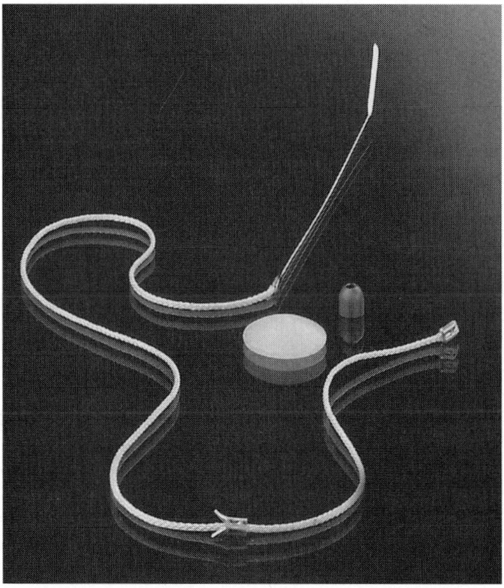

Fig. 3. Delponte's "harpoon tenorrhaphy." Two stab incisions are made 4 to 5 cm proximal to the rupture. The harpoon is passed through the proximal stump, the rupture site, and the distal stump by palpation, exiting through the skin either side of the calcaneum. The construct is tensioned through barbs proximally and lead crimps distally. The wire is removed after 6 weeks. (*Courtesy of* Fournitures Hospitalieres Industrie, Quimper, France; with permission.)

Johns revealed malaligned stumps in four out of five tendons repaired with the Ma and Griffith technique. For this reason, there have been efforts to devise a mini-open approach to Achilles tendon repair.

In 1995, Kakiuchi [22] published a report on a series of patients treated with a limited open and percutaneous repair. The stated aim of this new technique was to avoid the problems associated with a large incision, but to allow visualization of the tendon stumps, ensuring good approximation, which could not be achieved using a conventional percutaneous technique. A small incision is made over the palpable gap in the tendon and the tendon stumps are identified. A repair is then performed percutaneously, assisted by the use of two crude suture-passing devices fashioned from bent 2-mm Kirschner wires, which are passed beneath the paratenon (Fig. 4).

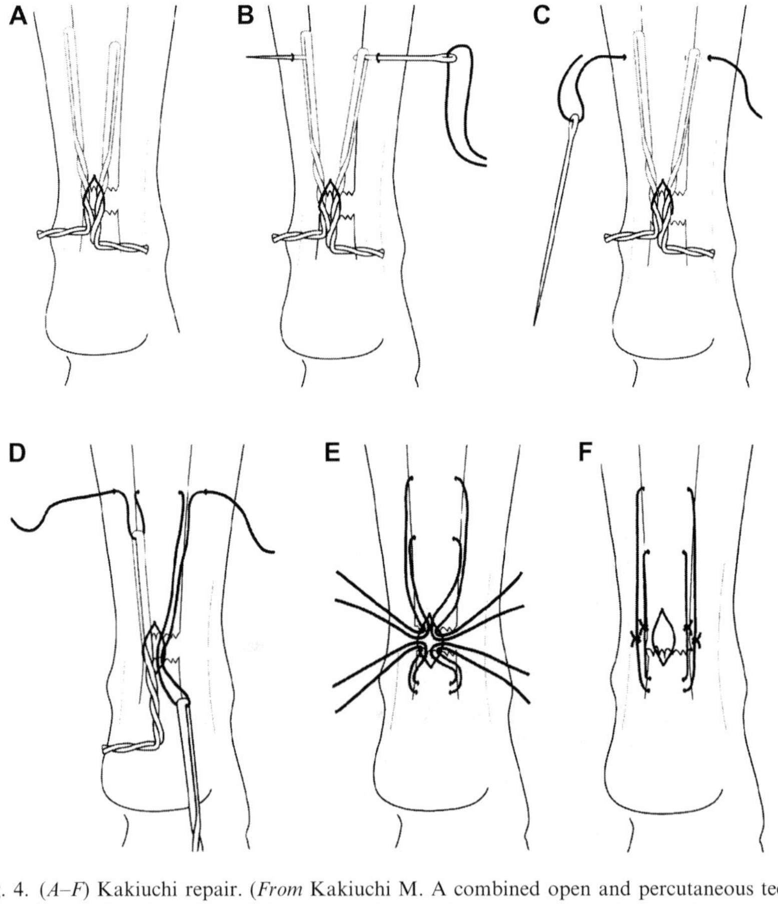

Fig. 4. (*A–F*) Kakiuchi repair. (*From* Kakiuchi M. A combined open and percutaneous technique for repair of tendo Achillis: comparison with open repair. J Bone Joint Surg Br 1995;77(1):61; with permission.)

In the report, Kakiuchi compared 12 patients treated by this new method with 10 patients treated with an open repair. The patients were reviewed at a mean interval of 5 years postsurgery. No recognized scoring system was used to assess the patients. Instead, the patients were interviewed and examined, recording both subjective and objective measures (symptoms, ability to return to sport, and hopping distance compared with the uninjured side). The results showed statistically significant better outcome in the combined open–percutaneous group. Kakiuchi's method was supported by the findings of a retrospective comparison of three groups of patients by Rebeccato and colleagues [24]. They compared open, percutaneous and combined mini-open plus percutaneous repairs in 52 patients. The outcomes measured were strength, performance, time of return to work, ankle range of motion, and calf circumference. They found that Kakiuchi's technique gave the best results.

Assal and colleagues [23] performed a cadaveric study to develop instrumentation for a system based on the principles of Kakiuchi's technique. They developed a guiding instrument, the design of which was based upon cadaveric findings of the shape (8° V angle) and cross-sectional area (81 mm^2) of the tendons of the cadaveric specimens (Fig. 5). The original instrument, made from stainless steel, is now also marketed as a single-use, rigid polymer device called Achillon (Integra Lifesciences Corporation, Plainsboro, New Jersey).

The Achillon system allows some degree of visual control at the repair site while enabling percutaneous passage of the sutures. The instrumentation theoretically lessens the likelihood of sural nerve entrapment because the sutures are retrieved by the inner arms of the device, which are placed beneath the paratenon layer. Only one small incision is made at the level of the rupture and the procedure can be performed under local anesthetic (Fig. 6).

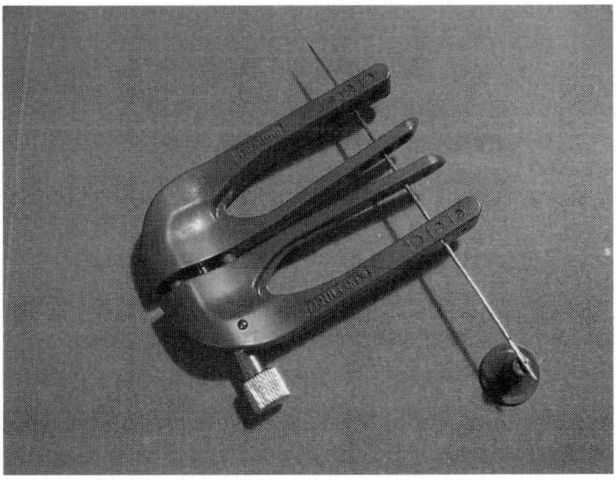

Fig. 5. The Achillon device.

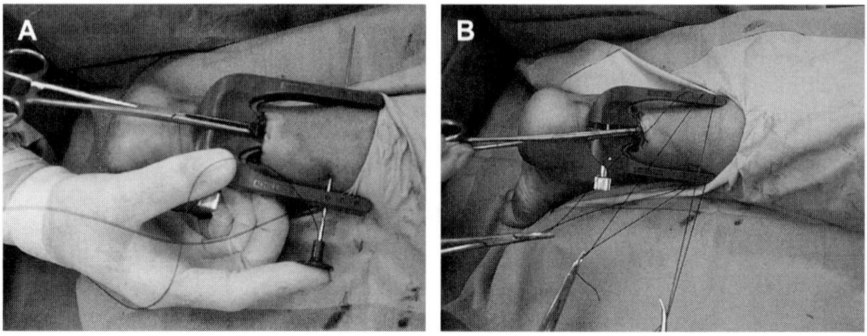

Fig. 6. (*A*) Passing suture. (*B*) Sutures in situ before removal of introducer.

Assal and colleagues report on a consecutive series of 87 patients treated with this device at three level-1 Swiss hospitals. Eighty-two patients were reviewed, of which 3 were excluded from the analysis. Each of these 3 had sustained early reruptures that the investigators felt were due to noncompliance with the postoperative regime in two cases and a fall from a bicycle in the third. The results revealed favorable American Orthopaedic Foot and Ankle Society (AOFAS) scores (mean 96 points) at an average 26-month follow-up. Isokinetic and endurance testing revealed no significant difference between the injured and uninjured sides and all patients returned to previous levels of sporting activity. There were no cases of wound infections or sural nerve disturbance. These promising results were replicated by Calder and Saxby [25] in a review of 46 patients treated with this technique. They modified the technique by recommending a small horizontal incision, suggesting that this may improve wound healing and cosmesis. They reported no reruptures; one superficial wound infection, which resolved with oral antibiotics; and 2 patients with transient sural nerve parasthesia. All patients were able to return to their previous sporting activities by 6 months, at which stage the mean AOFAS score was 98.4 (range 95–100). Ceccarelli and colleagues [26] prospectively studied two groups of patients, the first treated with a modified Ma and Griffith repair, the second with the Achillon. The modification of the Ma and Griffith's repair was to use two sutures rather than one and to place Bunnell constructs in each stump. Both groups were treated with the same semifunctional rehabilitation regime using a walker boot. The two groups were equivalent in terms of complications (no infections, no reruptures, no sural nerve injuries), AOFAS scores, and return to sports activity. The main limitation to the study was the small sample size (12 per group). Ismail and colleagues [27] have tested the in vitro strength of the Achillon repair. They compared matched groups of sheep Achilles tendons repaired with either the Achillon or a Kessler repair and tested them for mean load to failure. They found the Achillon to be a biomechanically sound method of repair with comparable tensile strength to a Kessler repair (153 ($N \pm 60$) versus 123 ($N \pm 24$)).

Summary

Treatment for repair of acute Achilles tendon rupture is slowly evolving but, as is the case with many areas of orthopaedic practice, a lack of prospective, randomized trials leaves a paucity of conclusive evidence to give a definitive answer as to the best treatment. There is certainly a role for percutaneous and mini-open techniques in treating the acutely ruptured tendo Achillis and some of the data available suggest that these techniques can give results equivalent to or better than those of an open repair, with the added benefit of fewer complications. Because there is less concern regarding wound healing in patients treated with this method, earlier mobilization may be allowed and studies have shown that early functional rehabilitation can increase the strength of healed tendons [28] and shorten rehabilitation time [29]. These finding have been backed up by a recent meta-analysis [30].

Khan and colleagues [1] have produced an important meta-analysis of the most methodologically sound studies published on this controversial topic. The investigators used rigorous methods for identification of appropriate studies and have clearly outlined their criteria for study inclusion and assessment of study quality. The methodological quality of each of the studies was scored out of 10 points. Despite the abundance of papers written on this topic in the literature, they could only find 12 worthy of inclusion. They have included 3 studies, amongst those 12 studies identified, with scores of 3 or 4 out of 10 and this may lead to criticism of skewing of the data [31]. They identified only 2 studies that compared percutaneous surgery with open surgery and that met their criteria. The conclusions they drew from the pooled data of these 2 studies were that both the rerupture rate and the infection rate were significantly lower in the percutaneous group.

More well-designed prospective randomized trials with large patient numbers are needed to give more conclusive evidence supporting one technique over the others.

References

[1] Khan R, Fick D, Keogh A, et al. Treatment of acute Achilles tendon ruptures. A meta-analysis of randomized, controlled trials. J Bone Joint Surg Am 2005;87:2202–10.

[2] Lo I, Kirkley A, Nonweiler B, et al. Operative versus nonoperative treatment of acute Achilles tendon ruptures: a quantitative review. Clin J Sport Med 1997;7(3):207–11.

[3] Lea R, Smith L. Rupture of the Achilles tendon. Nonsurgical treatment. Clin Orthop Relat Res 1968;60:115–8.

[4] Inglis AE, Scott WN, Sculco TP, et al. Ruptures of the tendo Achillis. An objective assessment of surgical and non-surgical treatment. J Bone Joint Surg Am 1976;58:990–3.

[5] Elliott A, Kennedy J, O'Malley M. Minimally invasive Achilles tendon repair using the Achillon repair system. Techniques in Foot and Ankle Surgery 2006;5(3):171–4.

[6] Carlstedt CA. Mechanical and chemical factors in tendon healing. Effects of indomethacin and surgery in the rabbit. Acta Orthop Scand Suppl 1987;224:1–75.

[7] Ma GWC, Griffith TG. Percutaneous repair of acute closed ruptured achilles tendon: a new technique. Clin Orthop Relat Res 1977;128:247–55.

[8] Klein W, Lang DM, Saleh M. The use of the Ma-Griffith technique for percutaneous repair of fresh ruptured tendo Achillis. Chir Organi Mov 1991;76(3):223–8.
[9] Hockenbury R, Johns J. A biomechanical in vitro comparison of open versus percutaneous repair of tendon Achilles. Foot Ankle 1990;11(2):67–72.
[10] Aktan Ikiz I, Ucerler H, Bilge O. The anatomic features of the sural nerve with an emphasis on its clinical importance. Foot Ankle Int 2005;26(7):560–7.
[11] Webb J, Moorjani N, Radford M. Anatomy of the sural nerve and its relation to the Achilles tendon. Foot Ankle Int 2000;21(6):475–7.
[12] Majewski M, Rohrbach M, Czaja S, et al. Avoiding sural nerve injuries during percutaneous Achilles tendon repair. Am J Sports Med 2006;34(5):793–8.
[13] Cretnik A, Zlapjpah L, Smrkolj V, et al. The strength of percutaneous methods of repair of the Achilles tendon: a biomechanical study. Med Sci Sports Exerc 2000;32(1):16–20.
[14] Cretnik A, Kasanovic M, Smrkolj V. Percutaneous versus open repair of the ruptured Achilles tendon: a comparative study. Am J Sports Med 2005;33(9):1369–79.
[15] Lim J, Dalal R, Waseem M. Percutaneous vs. open repair of the ruptured Achilles tendon—a prospective randomized controlled study. Foot Ankle Int 2001;22(7):559–68.
[16] Webb JM, Bannister GC. Percutaneous repair of the ruptured tendo Achillis. J Bone Joint Surg Br 1999;81(5):877–80.
[17] Wagnon R, Akayi M. The Webb–Bannister percutaneous technique for acute Achilles' tendon ruptures: a functional and MRI assessment. J Foot Ankle Surg 2005;44(6):437–44.
[18] Delponte P, Potier L, de Poulpiquet P, et al. [Treatment of subcutaneous ruptures of the Achilles tendon by percutaneous tenorrhaphy]. Rev Chir Orthop Reparatrice Appar Mot 1992;78(6):404–7 [in French].
[19] Maes R, Copin G, Averous C. Is percutaneous repair of the Achilles tendon a safe technique? A study of 124 cases. Acta Orthop Belg 2006;72(2):179–83.
[20] Gorschewsky O, Pitzl M, Putz A, et al. Percutaneous repair of the Achilles tendon. Foot Ankle Int 2004;25(4):219–24.
[21] Park H, Moon D, Yoon J. Limited open repair of ruptured Achilles tendons with Bunnel-type sutures. Foot Ankle Int 2001;22(12):985–7.
[22] Kakiuchi M. A combined open and percutaneous technique for repair of tendo Achillis: comparison with open repair. J Bone Joint Surg Br 1995;77(1):60–3.
[23] Assal M, Jung M, Stern R, et al. Limited open repair of Achilles tendon ruptures: a technique with a new instrument and findings of a prospective multicenter study. J Bone Joint Surg Am 2002;84(2):161–70.
[24] Rebeccato A, Santini S, Salmaso G, et al. Repair of the achilles tendon rupture: a functional comparison of three surgical techniques. J Foot Ankle Surg 2001;40(4):188–94.
[25] Calder JD, Saxby TS. Early, active rehabilitation following mini-open repair of Achilles tendon rupture: a prospective study. Br J Sports Med 2005;39(11):857–9.
[26] Ceccarelli F, Berti L, Giuriati L, et al. Percutaneous and minimally invasive techniques of Achilles tendon repair. Clin Orthop Relat Res 2007;458:188–93.
[27] Ismail M, Karim A, Calder J. The Achillon achilles tendon repair—is it strong enough? [abstract]. Presented at the EFORT Congress. Florence (Italy), May 11–15, 2007.
[28] Palmes D, Spiegel H, Schneider T, et al. Achilles tendon healing: long-term biomechanical effects of postoperative mobilization and immobilization in a new mouse model. J Orthop Res 2002;20(5):939–46.
[29] Maffulli N, Tallon C, Wong J, et al. Early weightbearing and ankle mobilization after open repair of acute midsubstance tears of the achilles tendon. Am J Sports Med 2003;31(5): 692–700.
[30] Suchak E, Spooner C, Reid D, et al. Postoperative rehabilitation protocols for Achilles tendon ruptures: a meta-analysis. Clin Orthop Relat Res 2006;445:216–21.
[31] McCormack RG. What treatment is most effective for acute Achilles tendon ruptures? Clin J Sport Med 2006;16(5):453–4.

ELSEVIER
SAUNDERS

Foot Ankle Clin N Am
12 (2007) 583–596

FOOT AND
ANKLE CLINICS

Chronic Rupture of Tendo Achillis

Nicola Maffulli, MD, MS, PhD, FRCS[a,*], Adam Ajis, MRCS[a], Umile Giuseppe Longo, MD[b], Vincenzo Denaro, MD[b]

[a]*Department of Trauma and Orthopaedic Surgery, Keele University School of Medicine, Thornburrow Drive, Hartshill, Stoke on Trent ST4 7QB Staffs, England, UK*
[b]*Department of Orthopaedic and Trauma Surgery, Campus Biomedico University, Via Longoni, 83 Rome, Italy*

The Achilles tendon is the most commonly ruptured tendon in the human body [1]. Complete rupture of the Achilles tendon can be experienced both by sedentary patients and athletes [1,2]. It is especially common in middle-aged men who occasionally participate in sport [3–6].

The definition of an old, chronic, or neglected rupture is variable. The most commonly used timeframe is 4 to 6 weeks from the time of injury [5,7–10]. Similarly, when there has been a delay in treatment, ruptures may be called chronic [10–15], neglected [7,14,16–20], or old [21,22].

Diagnosis is straightforward for experienced surgeons [23], and most Achilles tendon ruptures are promptly diagnosed [2,23,24]. Nevertheless, first-examining physicians may miss up to 20% of such injuries [25]. The diagnosis of chronic rupture can be more difficult [24,26] because, as fibrous scar tissue may have replaced the gap between the proximal and distal ends of the Achilles tendon, the gap palpable in acute ruptures is no longer present. There may also be less pain and swelling.

The management of chronic ruptures of tendo Achillis is usually different from that of acute rupture, as the tendon ends normally will have retracted. The blood supply to this area is poor, and the tendon ends have to be freshened to allow healing. Due to the increased gap, primary repair is not generally possible [24,26].

* Corresponding author.
E-mail address: n.maffulli@keele.ac.uk (N. Maffulli).

1083-7515/07/$ - see front matter
doi:10.1016/j.fcl.2007.07.007
foot.theclinics.com

Pathophysiology

Chronic ruptures of the Achilles tendon cause difficulty and impairment of plantar flexion [27]. The sheath may become thickened or adhere to the retracted tendon ends, and the gastrocnemius–soleus–Achilles-tendon complex acts as a weakened plantar flexor [27]. Often tendinous tissue is not present inside the sheath at the site of the defect because of tendon retraction [22]. The retracted tendon stumps are conically shaped proximally and bulbous distally [22]. The proximal tendon stump often adheres to the fascia posterior to the flexor hallucis longus muscle belly [28]. The tendon of plantaris, if present, may be hypertrophied. Thick scar tissue usually bridges the site of rupture [19,29–31] because of partial regeneration of the tendon [32]. Research involving rabbits has shown formations of well-organized connective tissue 56 days after calcaneal tendon resection. However, by 240 days, the tissue still did not display the fascicular arrangement of a tendon. This new tissue is weaker than a normal tendon and elongates with time [29,33]. Usually a gap is present between the tendon ends. The proximal stump is usually retracted, with shortening of the gastrocnemius–soleus complex and weakness of plantar flexion of the ankle. As the fiber shortens, the tension that the muscle fiber can produce decreases until it becomes zero when the fiber is approximately 60% of its resting length [34].

Diagnosis

Clinical examination

In acute ruptures, often a snapping sensation is felt in the posterior aspect of the ankle, with the patient then experiencing difficulty with weight-bearing on the affected side. There is often a palpable gap between the ruptured tendon ends [6]. The gap is most often 2 to 6 cm proximally from the insertion of the tendon. On average, the rupture site lies 4.78 cm proximal to the calcaneal insertion [35]. However, this may not be the case with chronic ruptures, which can prove more difficult to diagnose and manage [1,6,9,31,36–38].

Pain and swelling may have subsided for neglected or chronic rupture of the Achilles tendon, and the gap between the proximal and distal ends of the Achilles tendon may have filled with fibrous tissue [1,2,24]. Therefore, the gap between the tendon ends is less apparent or absent. Subtle evidence of pain and swelling around the proximal and distal stumps of the ruptured tendon may be present [12]. Active plantar flexion is also possible by the action tibialis posterior and the long toe flexors, contributing to a delayed diagnosis [13]. Active plantar flexion is, however, weak and associated with a limp [12]. A high index of suspicion is needed, and a range of special tests and investigations can be employed to aid accurate diagnosis.

Special tests

The calf-squeeze test is straightforward. It is often described as Thompson's or Simmonds' test [26], though Simmonds described the test 5 years before Thompson did. The patient lies prone on the examination couch with both feet hanging freely off the end. The examiner squeezes the proximal muscular half of the calf, avoiding direct pressure on the tendon. On the unaffected side, plantar flexion of the foot is evoked during the squeezing maneuver. On the ruptured side, no movement of the foot is noted during the squeezing maneuver.

Another simple, no-touch test is the Matles' test [39]. The patient lies prone on the examination table and is invited to flex both knees so that the tibiae come perpendicular to the floor. On the injured side, the angle between the anterior aspect of the shin and the dorsal aspect of the foot is more acute than on the uninjured side.

Simmonds' and Matles' tests are probably the two most common tests used to aid diagnosis, but O'Brien's [40] needle test or Copeland's sphygmomanometer test [41] can also be used. To perform the needle test, a hypodermic needle is inserted through the skin of the calf, approximately 0.5 cm off the midline and approximately 10 cm proximal to the insertion of the tendon. The needle should be inserted until its tip is just within the substance of the tendon. The ankle is then dorsiflexed and plantarflexed. If, on dorsiflexion, the needle points distally, the portion of the tendon distal to the needle is presumed to be intact. If the needle points proximally, there is presumed to be a loss of continuity between the needle and the site of insertion of the tendon [40].

In the sphygmomanometer test, a sphygmomanometer cuff is wrapped around the middle of the calf with the patient lying prone. The cuff is inflated to 100 mm Hg (13.3 kPa) with the foot in plantar flexion. The foot is then dorsiflexed. If the pressure rises to around 140 mm Hg (18.7 kPa), the tendo Achillis unit is presumed to be intact. If the pressure remains at or around 100 mm Hg, the patient likely has a tendo Achillis rupture. If two of the above tests are positive, the diagnosis of Achilles tendon rupture is certain [2].

Imaging

At lateral radiographs of the ankle, the Kager's triangle [42] (a triangular fat-filled space between the anterior aspect of the Achilles tendon, the posterior aspect of the tibia, and the superior aspect of the calcaneus) looses its configuration and can be distorted if there is a rupture. Also, deformation of the distal tendon contours from loss of tone can be seen [31]. Radiographs assist by ruling out a calcaneal avulsion and prior foot and ankle difficulties [13]. In a series of chronic tendo Achillis ruptures, calcification in the distal portion of the proximal stump of the Achilles tendon was present in three of seven patients [12]. Additionally attritional changes due to old athletic injuries are often apparent on plain radiograph [13].

Real-time high-resolution ultrasonography is an inexpensive, rapid, and dynamic diagnostic aid [43]. It is user dependent, and may require substantial experience to operate the probe and interpret the images correctly [44–47]. High-frequency probes provide the best results [47]. A normal Achilles tendon appears as a hypoechogenic, ribbon-like image contained within two hyperechogenic bands that are separated when the tendon is relaxed and more compact when the tendon is under tension. When the Achilles tendon ruptures, an ultrasound scan reveals an acoustic vacuum with thick irregular edges (Fig. 1) [45].

The multiplanar imaging capabilities of MRI combined with its excellent soft tissue contrast characteristics make it ideally suited for imaging of the rupture of the Achilles tendon. In the evaluation of the Achilles tendon, sagittal and axial planes, using combinations of T1- and T2-weighted imaging sequences, are most useful. MRI allows determination of the extent and nature of the condition of the tendon ends in complete Achilles tendon tears [48]. Subtle thickness changes are detected in the axial plane and the longitudinal extent of the tear on sagittal images. A normal Achilles tendon is viewed as an area of low signal intensity on all sequences. The tendon tapers smoothly and shows no focal defects. The dark band of the tendon is well contrasted from the high signal intensity of the pre-Achilles fat pad [48]. Any high signal intratendinous intensity is viewed as abnormal [48]. For a T1-weighted image, a complete rupture is visualized as disruption of the signal within the tendon, mixed with hemorrhage and edema that localizes in the pre-Achilles fat pad. Older complete tears display hemorrhage as low signal intensity on T1-weighted images. A T2 image will show generalized increased signal intensity representing the edema and hemorrhage within and around the ruptured tendon [41]. Discontinuity, fraying of the tendon, widening of the tendon edges, abnormal orientation and condition of the fibers, and retraction of the tendon edges into the calf are more comprehensively seen on T2 [41].

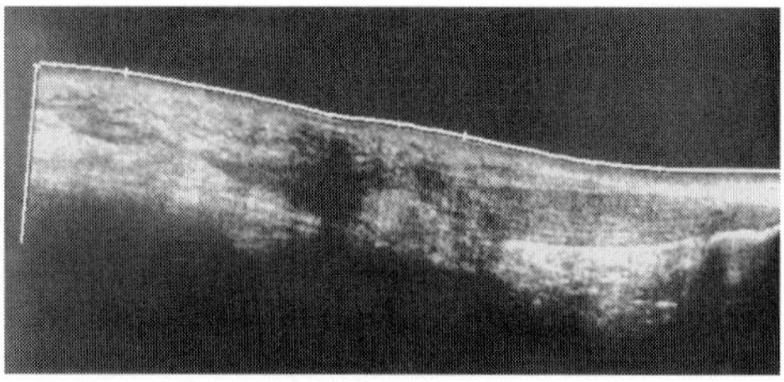

Fig. 1. Ultrasound scan of a chronic tear of the Achilles tendon. There is loss of definition of the tendo Achillis, with a large hypoechoic area seen in the tendon itself. This corresponds to the retracted tendon stumps.

Injury guidelines and classification with a view to treatment

Both Myerson [29] and Kuwada [44] have noted that the size of the Achilles tendon defect is likely to affect management.

Myerson [29] treats ruptures of the Achilles tendon based on the size of tendon defect:

- Defects of 1 to 2 cm are treated with end-to-end anastomosis and posterior compartment fasciotomy.
- Defects between 2 and 5 cm are repaired using V-Y lengthening, occasionally augmented with a tendon transfer.
- Defects greater than 5 cm are repaired using tendon transfer alone or in combination with V-Y advancement.
- Due to the bulk of the tendon at the point it is passed inferiorly, Myerson prefers not to use a turndown flap, but acknowledges it does have a role.

Kuwada [44] grades Achilles tendon injuries I to IV:

- Type I injuries are classified as partial tears treated with cast immobilization.
- Type II injuries are complete ruptures with a defect up to 3 cm. These are treated with end-to-end anastomosis.
- Type III injuries have a 3- to 6-cm defect after debridement of the proximal and distal ends of the Achilles tendon to healthy tissue. This grade of defect requires a tendon graft flap, possibly augmented with synthetic graft.
- Type IV injury is a defect that is greater than 6 cm and requires gastrocnemius recession, a free tendon graft, and/or synthetic graft.

Kuwada's [44] classification scheme for tendo Achilles rupture is based on 28 repairs and 102 gastrocnemius recessions.

Management

The management of chronic and neglected rupture of the Achilles tendon is usually different from that of acute rupture, as the tendon ends have retracted. The blood supply to this area is poor.

Surgery requires the tendon edges to be freshened, and, as they will be retracted, a large gap will thus be produced. Due to the increased gap, primary repair may be difficult [24]. Various techniques have been described to bridge the gap. Subsequently, the repair requires reinforcement (augmentation) through the use of a turndown flap, a tendon transfer, a tendon graft, or synthetic materials [12–15,49].

Nonoperative management

Christensen [50] reported a series of neglected ruptures treated conservatively. Eighteen of 51 patients with 57 ruptures (nearly two thirds of which were neglected) were treated conservatively. For 7 patients, conservative management was chosen because the operation was contraindicated or refused. For 11 patients, conservative treatment was chosen because the rupture was several months old and the triceps surae showed signs of regaining strength. For those 11, the injury was managed "expectantly." Satisfactory results (ie, normal gait, return to previous occupation, and slight or no discomfort) were obtained in 10 of 18 (56%) of nonoperated patients. In addition, Christensen reported that improvement in all nonoperated cases occurs slowly, sometimes over several years. Brace management should be considered in patients without functional deficit and in those with potential wound-healing problems or anesthetic contraindications to surgery. A brace or ankle–foot orthosis was also reported as beneficial [29].

Operative management

V-Y tendinous flap

The procedure for using a V-Y tendinous flap was reported by Abraham and Pankovich [49] and is applicable to neglected, chronic ruptures of the Achilles tendon. The aim of this procedure is to achieve end-to-end anastomosis of the Achilles tendon. This is made possible by a sliding tendinous flap developed over the proximal portion of the tendon, by making an inverted V incision, which is then repaired in a Y fashion. Abraham and Pankovich [49] reported four patients, with three of the patients regaining full strength of the triceps surae muscle and able to raise their heels from the floor equally when on tiptoe. One patient continued to complain of slight weakness of the triceps surae muscle, and the heel-to-floor distance on the operated side was 2 cm less than on the operated side. The only complication was one sural nerve neuroma. Leitner and colleagues [21] reported three patients with tendon defects of 9 to 10 cm managed successfully using this technique. Kissel and colleagues [30] used the same technique, augmented with plantaris weave-and-pullout suture in 14 patients. Parker and Repinecz [51] described a similar technique in which a tongue-in-groove advancement of gastrocnemius aponeurosis was used to close a 6.5-cm defect in one patient. They reported this as easier than V-Y advancement, and up to 50% more length can be accomplished.

Turndown flaps

Fascial turndown flaps can be used for an anatomic repair of chronic rupture of tendo Achillis. This technique accommodates a stronger suture line and results in fewer adhesions between sutured site and skin.

Christensen [50] and Gerhardt [52] separately described similar techniques. After suturing the tendon ends, they raised a distally based flap from the gastrocnemius aponeurosis, turned it over itself across the suture line, and sutured to the distal part of the Achilles tendon. Silfverskiold [53] twisted the gastrocnemius flap through 180° before suturing it distally. This resulted in the smooth surface of the flap coming in contact with the skin, thereby decreasing the chance of adhesion between the flap itself and the overlying tissue. Toygar [54] described a technique for chronic ruptures where continuity between the two ends is difficult to regain. The gap is bridged by two flaps raised from the two ends of the tendon, one from medial side and the other from the lateral side. Weisbach [55] described another technique to address the same problem. Along with the gastrocnemius flap, he raised another flap from the distal stump of the Achilles tendon, and sutured these two flaps to bridge the gap.

Rush's [19] operation to reconstruct a neglected rupture of the tendo Achilles uses the aponeurosis of the gastrocnemius–soleus muscle fashioned into a tube. The repair was felt to be strong and effective, and produced good results in five patients. Bosworth [33] reported on seven patients, five of whom with chronic ruptures. He used a strip of the superficial part of the tendinous portion of the proximal stump of the Achilles tendon to augment the repair. He made a posterior longitudinal incision and dissected a 0.5-in by 7- to 9-in strip of tendon on a distal pedicle. He then threaded the strip of tendon through the trimmed ends of the ruptured tendon and sutured it to the trimmed tendon ends with the foot in plantarflexion. No complications occurred. Other investigators have used V-Y advancement and flap turndown in combination [20] or as isolated techniques [56] with good results.

Peroneus brevis transfer

Peroneus brevis tendon transfer for rupture of the Achilles tendon was popularized by Perez-Teuffer [57]. In the original technique, the peroneus brevis tendon was passed through a transosseous drill hole in the calcaneum. The ruptures in this series were acute, with 28 of 30 patients able to return to their original level of sport. Turco and Spinella [13] augmented end-to-end repair of the Achilles tendon, with a modification of Teuffer's technique, by passing peroneus brevis through the distal tendon stump rather than through the calcaneus. McClelland and Maffulli [24] approach the Achilles tendon medially, and deliver the Achilles tendon through the posteromedial wound. The distally transsected peroneal tendon is gently pulled through the inferior peroneal retinaculum. Thus the blood supply is retained from the intermuscular septum. The peroneus brevis tendon is then woven through the ends of the ruptured Achilles tendon, passing through small coronal incisions in the distal stump, and then through similar incisions in the proximal stump (Figs. 2 and 3). The tendon of plantaris, if present, can also be harvested to augment the repair if there is a large gap. As peroneus brevis is used to reconstruct the Achilles tendon, the peroneus longus becomes the sole evertor of the foot, and continues to maintain the transverse arch. Gallant and colleagues [58] assessed eversion and plantar flexion strength after repair of Achilles tendon rupture using peroneus brevis tendon transfer and found mild objective eversion and plantar flexion weakness. However, subjective assessment revealed no functional compromise [58]. Also, if the tendon of peroneus brevis is placed distally in a

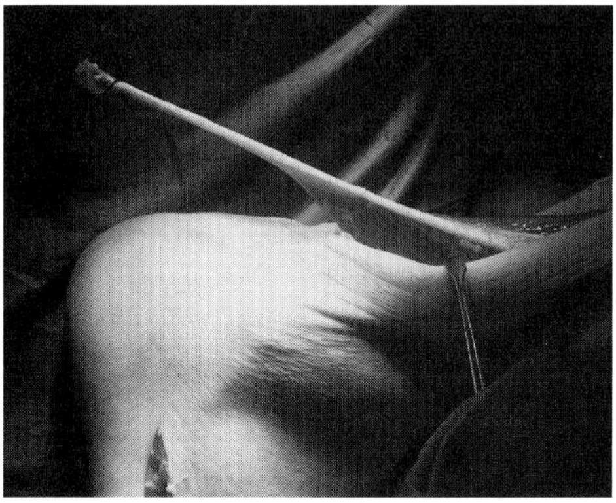

Fig. 2. Reconstruction of a chronic tear of the Achilles tendon using the tendon of peroneus brevis.

lateral-to-medial direction, it does not duplicate the medial pull of a normal Achilles tendon [12].

Flexor digitorum longus

Mann and colleagues [12] described a technique using the flexor digitorum longus as a graft in seven patients. He used a medial hockey stick incision for the Achilles tendon, and a second medial incision on the foot inferior and distal to the navicular extending toward the first metatarsophalangeal joint to allow access to the flexor digitorum longus. The flexor digitorum longus was then cut proximally to its division into separate digital branches. The distal stump was sutured to the adjacent flexor hallucis longus. The proximal stump of the flexor digitorum longus was delivered into the wound. They also included a proximal fascial turndown flap in all cases and, when length allowed, the proximal stump was reattached to the calcaneus with a pullout technique. Six of the seven patients had an excellent result, and one a fair result. There were no reruptures at an average follow-up of 39 months.

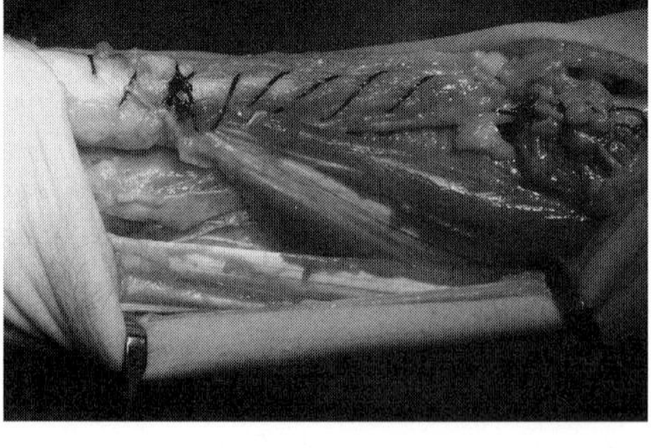

Fig. 3. Reconstruction of a chronic tear of the Achilles tendon using the tendon of peroneus brevis.

Flexor hallucis longus

The flexor hallucis longus has a long tendon (10–12 cm) that allows bridging large tendo Achillis defects. When transferred, it also maintains the normal muscle balance of the ankle because a plantar flexor is transferred to a plantar flexor. However, in athletic patients, the loss of push-off strength from the hallux causes difficulty when sprinting [24]. Wapner and colleagues [14] showed in seven patients that flexor hallucis longus could be used as a graft. Once the flexor hallucis longus was harvested, Wapner and colleagues passed the tendon through a drill hole in the calcaneum, and wove it through the ruptured ends of the tendo Achillis. The distal end of the tendon of the flexor hallucis longus was tenodesed to the tendon of the flexor digitorum longus to the second toe. Three patients had an excellent result, three had a good result, and one a fair result (level 4 evidence). All patients developed a functionally insignificant range-of-movement loss at the ankle and hallux. Cybex testing revealed a 29.5% reduction in plantar flexion power compared with the normal side. No functional disability was noted secondary to flexor hallucis longus harvest. This is in agreement with Frenette and Jackson [59], who reported 10 cases of flexor hallucis longus tendon laceration in young athletes, 4 of which were not repaired, with no disability evident. A flexor hallucis longus transfer has several theoretical advantages:

The long durable tendon has a stronger muscle than that for other tendon transfers [3].

The axis of flexor hallucis longus contraction closely reproduces that of the Achilles tendon.

The flexor hallucis longus fires in phase with the gastrocnemius–soleus muscle.

The anatomic proximity makes the surgical technique easier and avoids the need to disturb the neurovascular bundle or lateral compartment muscles.

Harvesting of flexor hallucis longus allows maintenance of normal muscle balance of the ankle (ie, plantar flexor to plantar flexor).

Finally, this technique adds 10 to 12 cm of tendon compared with Hansen's technique, allowing weaving of the tendon through the Achilles. This technique is similar to that used by Dalal and Zenios [11], who reported excellent results following reconstruction of three chronic ruptures in two elderly patients. Wilcox and colleagues [15] treated 20 patients with chronic Achilles tendinopathy, with a similar technique.

Gracilis

Maffulli and Leadbetter [28] used the tendon of gracilis as a free graft to bridge the gap in chronic ruptures of the Achilles tendon. If, after trying to reduce the gap of the ruptured Achilles tendon, the gap is still greater than 6 cm despite maximal plantar flexion of the ankle and traction on the Achilles tendon stumps, the gracilis tendon is harvested with a tendon stripper.

When present, the tendon of plantaris can be harvested with the tendon stripper, left attached distally, and used to reinforce the reconstruction (Figs. 4 and 5) [28]. Two patients were classified as having an excellent result, and 15 of 21 patients achieved a good result.

Synthetic materials

The use of synthetic materials to repair Achilles tendon rupture present advantages in that the technique is relatively simple and there is no donor site morbidity. However, specific problems and complications can arise, such as infections.

Howard and colleagues [60] used carbon fiber to repair five neglected ruptures. After a follow-up period from 4 to 19 months, the average plantar flexion strength was 88% compared with the opposite limb. All patients had excellent results, but some complications resulted with stiffness in two patients and one delayed wound-healing. Parsons and colleagues [61] used an absorbable polymer carbon fiber composite ribbon in 48 patients with Achilles tendon ruptures, 27 of which were chronic. The ribbon was woven through the proximal and distal stumps with six to eight passes to bridge the defect. A proximal tendon flap was used "at the surgeon's discretion." From their own devised score, 86% had a good or excellent result. Twenty-nine of the original 48 patients had at least 1-year follow-up and it is unknown if these were for acute or chronic ruptures. Complications included two reruptures, two deep infections, and three superficial infections. Investigations have been performed on carbon fiber in sheep tendons [62]. Carbon fiber fragmentation has been shown in sheep calcaneal tendons associated with

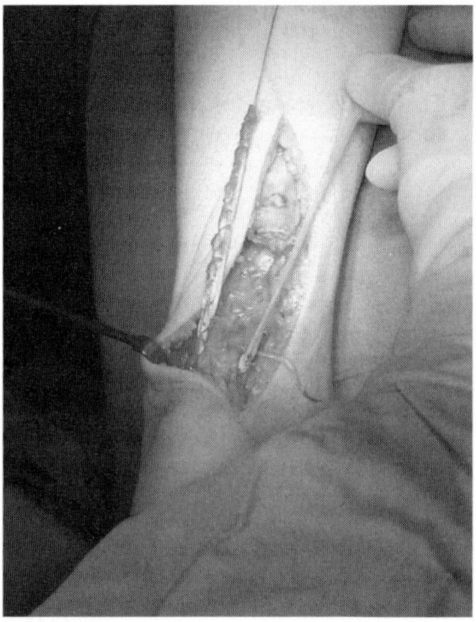

Fig. 4. Reconstruction of a chronic tear of the Achilles tendon using the tendon of gracilis.

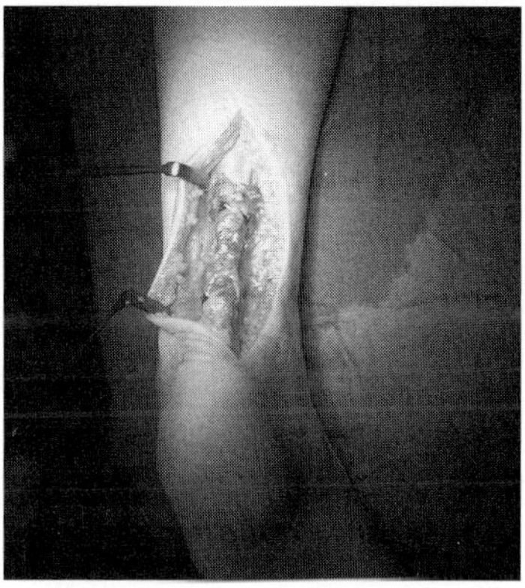

Fig. 5. Reconstruction of a chronic tear of the Achilles tendon using the tendon of gracilis.

a poor collagen response. With polyester implants, the neotendon was denser, more collagenous, and closely adherent [62].

Ozaki and colleagues [18] used three layers of Marlex mesh (polypropylene) to reconstruct neglected ruptures. The gaps ranged between 5 and 12 cm in a series of six patients. The minimum follow-up in this series was 2.4 years, with all patients showing satisfactory function and averaging 94% plantar flexion strength compared with the uninjured side. No complications were noted in the series (level 4 evidence).

Dacron vascular grafts have been used to augment Achilles tendon rupture [63,64], and have shown good or excellent results in acute rupture (level 4 evidence).

Jennings and Sefton [10] used polyester tape with a Bunnel-type suture in 16 chronic ruptures. The tape was tensioned so the ankle could just dorsiflex to neutral. One patient required removal of the tape from around the calcaneum, 1 had a sural nerve injury, and 3 had superficial wound infections. No reruptures occurred (level 4 evidence).

Fascia lata

Using fascia lata to repair and augment Achilles tendon rupture has produced good results [17,22,27]. Bugg and Boyd [16] reported 21 Achilles tendon ruptures or lacerations, 10 of which were chronic. They bridged the gap in the Achilles tendon with three strips of fascia lata, with a sheet of fascia lata sutured around these grafts in a tube-like fashion, with the serosal surface outwards and the seam placed anteriorly and sutured to the proximal distal stumps. A wire pullout suture was also used. No formal results were given, but two case reports were provided stating that the technique has produced satisfactory functional and cosmetic results.

Allografts

Repair using allografts is not commonly reported on in the literature and, as in the case of synthetic materials, does not require a donor site. Nellas and colleagues [65] used two strips of freeze-dried tendo Achillis allograft to reconstruct a 4.5-cm tendon defect, following debridement of an infected primary repair. The patient had a good functional result, although had lower peak torque compared with the uninjured side.

Haraguchi and colleagues [66] used Achilles tendon allograft for both chronic rupture and extensive tendinosis. The cortical bone in this procedure is removed from the patient's heel allowing room for the allograft, which is secured in position with two 4.0-mm screws. The graft is then tensioned and repaired to the native Achilles tendon. No formal results have been published as yet for this series, but no rejection of allograft has been observed and no transmission of disease to the host has occurred.

Summary

Chronic ruptures of tendo Achillis are uncommon but potentially debilitating. The choice of management is partly guided by the size of the tendon defect with the optimal management being surgical. There are many different techniques that can be used to repair or reconstruct the rupture. Comparison of different techniques is difficult because relevant studies tend to be retrospective and small. Every patient is different, and can present with varied comorbidity, varied time of presentation, and different lengths of Achilles tendon retraction gap. Management should be tailored to the individual. Tissue engineering technology shows promise, but is in its infancy and its application in clinical studies is probably still far away. Further research and clinical trials are needed to evaluate its efficacy in humans.

References

[1] Maffulli N. Rupture of the Achilles tendon. J Bone Joint Surg Am 1999;81:1019–36.

[2] Maffulli N. The clinical diagnosis of subcutaneous tear of the Achilles tendon. A prospective study in 174 patients. Am J Sports Med 1998;26:266–70.

[3] Silver RL, de la Garza J, Rang M. The myth of muscle balance. A study of relative strengths and excursions of normal muscles about the foot and ankle. J Bone Joint Surg Br 1985;67:432–7.

[4] Puddu G, Ippolito E, Postacchini F. A classification of Achilles tendon disease. Am J Sports Med 1976;4:145–50.

[5] Boyden EM, Kitaoka HB, Cahalan TD, et al. Late versus early repair of Achilles tendon rupture. Clinical and biomechanical evaluation. Clin Orthop Relat Res 1995;317:150–8.

[6] Hattrup SJ, Johnson KA. A review of ruptures of the Achilles tendon. Foot Ankle 1985;6:34–8.

[7] Gabel S, Manoli A 2nd. Neglected rupture of the Achilles tendon. Foot Ankle Int 1994;15:512–7.

[8] Gillespie HS, George EA. Results of surgical repair of spontaneous rupture of the Achilles tendon. J Trauma 1969;9:247–9.

[9] Inglis AE, Scott WN, Sculco TP, et al. Ruptures of the tendo Achillis. An objective assessment of surgical and non-surgical treatment. J Bone Joint Surg Am 1976;58:990–3.

[10] Jennings AG, Sefton GK. Chronic rupture of tendo Achillis. Long-term results of operative management using polyester tape. J Bone Joint Surg Br 2002;84:361–3.

[11] Dalal RB, Zenios M. The flexor hallucis longus tendon transfer for chronic tendo-Achilles ruptures revisited. Ann R Coll Surg Engl 2003;85:283.
[12] Mann RA, Holmes GB Jr, Seale KS, et al. Chronic rupture of the Achilles tendon: a new technique of repair. J Bone Joint Surg Am 1991;73:214–9.
[13] Turco VJ, Spinella AJ. Achilles tendon ruptures—peroneus brevis transfer. Foot Ankle 1987;7:253–9.
[14] Wapner KL, Pavlock GS, Hecht PJ, et al. Repair of chronic Achilles tendon rupture with flexor hallucis longus tendon transfer. Foot Ankle 1993;14:443–9.
[15] Wilcox DK, Bohay DR, Anderson JG. Treatment of chronic achilles tendon disorders with flexor hallucis longus tendon transfer/augmentation. Foot Ankle Int 2000;21:1004–10.
[16] Bugg EI Jr, Boyd BM. Repair of neglected rupture or laceration of the Achilles tendon. Clin Orthop Relat Res 1968;56:73–5.
[17] Tobin WJ. Repair of the neglected ruptured and severed Achilles tendon. Am Surg 1953;19: 514–22.
[18] Ozaki J, Fujiki J, Sugimoto K, et al. Reconstruction of neglected Achilles tendon rupture with Marlex mesh. Clin Orthop Relat Res 1989;238:204–8.
[19] Rush JH. Operative repair of neglected rupture of the tendo Achillis. Aust N Z J Surg 1980; 50:420–2.
[20] Us AK, Bilgin SS, Aydin T, et al. Repair of neglected Achilles tendon ruptures: procedures and functional results. Arch Orthop Trauma Surg 1997;116:408–11.
[21] Leitner A, Voigt C, Rahmanzadeh R. Treatment of extensive aseptic defects in old Achilles tendon ruptures: methods and case reports. Foot Ankle 1992;13:176–80.
[22] Zadek I. Repair of old rupture of the tendo-Achilles by means of fascia. Report of a case. J Bone Joint Surg 1940;22:1070–1.
[23] DiStefano VJ, Nixon JE. Achilles tendon rupture: pathogenesis, diagnosis, and treatment by a modified pullout wire technique. J Trauma 1972;12:671–7.
[24] McClelland D, Maffulli N. Neglected rupture of the Achilles tendon: reconstruction with peroneus brevis tendon transfer. Surgeon 2004;2:209–13.
[25] Maffulli N. Clinical tests in sports medicine: more on Achilles tendon. Br J Sports Med 1996; 30:250.
[26] Simmonds FA. The diagnosis of the ruptured Achilles tendon. Practitioner 1957;179:56–8.
[27] Platt H. Observation of some tendon repairs. Br Med J 1931;1:611–5.
[28] Mafulli N, Leadbetter WB. Free gracilis tendon graft in neglected tears of the Achilles tendon. Clin J Sport Med 2005;15(2):56–61.
[29] Myerson MS. Achilles tendon ruptures. Instr Course Lect 1999;48:219–30.
[30] Kissel CG, Blacklidge DK, Crowley DL. Repair of neglected Achilles tendon ruptures—procedure and functional results. J Foot Ankle Surg 1994;33:46–52.
[31] Arner O, Lindholm A, Orell SR. Histologic changes in subcutaneous rupture of the Achilles tendon; a study of 74 cases. Acta Chir Scand 1959;116:484–90.
[32] Conway AM, Dorner RW, Zuckner J. Regeneration of resected calcaneal tendon of the rabbit. Anat Rec 1967;158:43–9.
[33] Bosworth DM. Repair of defects in the tendo Achillis. J Bone Joint Surg Am 1956;38-A:111–4.
[34] Elftman H. Biomechanics of muscle with particular application to studies of gait. J Bone Joint Surg Am 1966;48:363–77.
[35] Krueger-Franke M, Siebert CH, Scherzer S. Surgical treatment of ruptures of the Achilles tendon: a review of long-term results. Br J Sports Med 1995;29:121–5.
[36] Carden DG, Noble J, Chalmers J, et al. Rupture of the calcaneal tendon. The early and late management. J Bone Joint Surg Br 1987;69:416–20.
[37] Ballas MT, Tytko J, Mannarino F. Commonly missed orthopedic problems. Am Fam Physician 1998;57:267–74.
[38] Nestorson J, Movin T, Moller M, et al. Function after Achilles tendon rupture in the elderly: 25 patients older than 65 years followed for 3 years. Acta Orthop Scand 2000;71:64–8.

[39] Matles AL. Rupture of the tendo Achilles. Another diagnostic sign. Bull Hosp Joint Dis 1975;36:48–51.
[40] O'Brien T. The needle test for complete rupture of the Achilles tendon. J Bone Joint Surg Am 1984;66:1099–101.
[41] Copeland SA. Rupture of the Achilles tendon: a new clinical test. Ann R Coll Surg Engl 1990;72:270–1.
[42] Kager H. Zur klinikund. Diagnostik des Achillessehnenrisses. Chirurg 1939;11:691–5.
[43] Popovic N, Lemaire R. Diagnosis and treatment of acute ruptures of the Achilles tendon. Current concepts review. Acta Orthop Belg 1999;65:458–71.
[44] Kuwada GT. Classification of tendo Achillis rupture with consideration of surgical repair techniques. J Foot Surg 1990;29:361–5.
[45] Maffulli N, Regine R, Angelillo M, et al. Ultrasound diagnosis of Achilles tendon pathology in runners. Br J Sports Med 1987;21:158–62.
[46] Crass JR, van de Vegte GL, Harkavy LA. Tendon echogenicity: ex vivo study. Radiology 1988;167:499–501.
[47] Fornage BD. Achilles tendon: US examination. Radiology 1986;159:759–64.
[48] Kabbani YM, Mayer DP. Magnetic resonance imaging of tendon pathology about the foot and ankle. Part I. Achilles tendon. J Am Podiatr Med Assoc 1993;83:418–20.
[49] Abraham E, Pankovich AM. Neglected rupture of the Achilles tendon. Treatment by V-Y tendinous flap. J Bone Joint Surg Am 1975;57:253–5.
[50] Christensen I. Rupture of the Achilles tendon; analysis of 57 cases. Acta Chir Scand 1953; 106:50–60.
[51] Parker RG, Repinecz M. Neglected rupture of the achilles tendon. Treatment by modified Strayer gastrocnemius recession. J Am Podiatry Assoc 1979;69:548–55.
[52] Gerhardt K. Zur wiederherstellungschirurgie. Versorgung des Achillessenenrisses. Archiv Klinische Chirurgie 1937;189:681–93.
[53] Silfverskiold F. Uber die subkutane totale Achillesschnenruptur und deren behandlung. Acta Chir Scand 1941;84:393–401.
[54] Toygar O. Subkutane Ruptur der Achillesschne. Helvet Chir Acta 1947;14:209–31.
[55] Weisbach K. Betriebe in den risen der Achillessehnerisses. [Reconstructive operations in lacerations of Achilles tendon]. Wien Med Wochenschr 1954;104:361–4.
[56] Barnes MJ, Hardy AE. Delayed reconstruction of the calcaneal tendon. J Bone Joint Surg Br 1986;68:121–4.
[57] Perez-Teuffer A. Traumatic rupture of the Achilles tendon. Reconstruction by transplant and graft using the lateral peroneus brevis. Orthop Clin North Am 1974;5:89–93.
[58] Gallant GG, Massie C, Turco VJ. Assessment of eversion and plantar flexion strength after repair of Achilles tendon rupture using peroneus brevis tendon transfer. Am J Orthop 1995;24:257–61.
[59] Frenette JP, Jackson DW. Lacerations of the flexor hallucis longus in the young athlete. J Bone Joint Surg Am 1977;59:673–6.
[60] Howard CB, Winston I, Bell W, et al. Late repair of the calcaneal tendon with carbon fibre. J Bone Joint Surg Br 1984;66:206–8.
[61] Parsons JR, Weiss AB, Schenk RS, et al. Long-term follow-up of Achilles tendon repair with an absorbable polymer carbon fiber composite. Foot Ankle 1989;9:179–84.
[62] Amis AA, Campbell JR, Kempson SA, et al. Comparison of the structure of neotendons induced by implantation of carbon or polyester fibres. J Bone Joint Surg Br 1984;66:131–9.
[63] Levy M, Velkes S, Goldstein J, et al. A method of repair for Achilles tendon ruptures without cast immobilization. Preliminary report. Clin Orthop Relat Res 1984;187:199–204.
[64] Lieberman JR, Lozman J, Czajka J, et al. Repair of Achilles tendon ruptures with Dacron vascular graft. Clin Orthop Relat Res 1988;234:204–8.
[65] Nellas ZJ, Loder BG, Wertheimer SJ. Reconstruction of an Achilles tendon defect utilizing an Achilles tendon allograft. J Foot Ankle Surg 1996;35:144–8 [discussion: 190].
[66] Haraguchi N, Bluman EM, Myerson MS. Reconstruction of chronic Achilles tendon disorders with Achilles tendon allograft. Techniques in Foot and Ankle Surgery 2005;4:154–9.

ELSEVIER
SAUNDERS

Foot Ankle Clin N Am
12 (2007) 597–615

FOOT AND
ANKLE CLINICS

Management of Insertional Tendinopathy of the Achilles Tendon

Matthew Solan, FRCS (Tr&Orth)[a,b,c,*], Mark Davies, FRCS (Tr&Orth)[a]

[a]*London Foot and Ankle Centre, Hospital of St. John and St. Elizabeth, 60 Grove End Road, London NW8 9NH, UK*
[b]*Department of Orthopaedic Surgery, Royal Surrey County Hospital, Guildford, Surrey, GU2 7XX, UK*
[c]*Surrey Foot and Ankle Clinic, Guildford Nuffield Hospital, Stirling Road, Guildford, Surrey, GU2 7RF, UK*

Heel pain is a common complaint and is often poorly managed. Nonoperative treatments are highly effective for the vast majority of patients, and surgery is reserved for recalcitrant cases. Both operative and nonoperative treatments can be selected most appropriately if a full assessment of the patient has resulted in an accurate diagnosis.

The first distinction to make clinically is between plantar heel pain and posterior heel pain. The former is commonly caused by plantar fasciitis. Other orthopaedic causes include a stress fracture of the os calcis or, less commonly, tarsal tunnel syndrome. Inflammatory and rare neoplastic pathologies must be borne in mind, especially if first-line treatments fail to improve symptoms (Box 1).

Posterior heel pain most commonly arises from the Achilles tendon. Clain and Baxter [1] classified Achilles pain as arising from the insertional portion of the tendon or from the noninsertional region. This distinction is helpful clinically.

Noninsertional Achilles tendon pathology is more common than insertional tendinopathy and is due to degeneration within the substance of the tendon, thickening of the paratenon, or a combination of the two. Noninsertional tendinopathy will not be discussed further in this article.

Sever's disease affects children and is best considered as a traction apophysitis. Activity modification is the mainstay of treatment for these

* Corresponding author. London Foot and Ankle Centre, Hospital of St. John and St. Elizabeth, 60 Grove End Road, London NW8 9NH, United Kingdom.
E-mail address: matthewsolan1@aol.com (M. Solan).

doi:10.1016/j.fcl.2007.07.005

Box 1. Differential diagnosis of heel pain

Posterior heel pain
Insertional tendinopathy
Retrocalcaneal bursitis
Pump bumps
Os trigonum
Flexor hallucis longus
Gout
Seronegative arthropathy

Plantar heel pain
Plantar fasciitis
Os calcis stress fracture
Tarsal tunnel syndrome
Rheumatoid arthritis
Infection (especially in diabetics)

young patients, who are usually highly active in sports. An orthotic to lift the heel may be of benefit and casting is seldom required [2]. Sever's disease is a self-limiting condition. It will not be covered here in more detail.

Semantics in Achilles tendon pain

Maffulli [3–6] proposed a logical and easy-to-use nomenclature for describing Achilles tendon pathologies (Box 2). This has reduced the use of many confusing synonyms that were previously seen in the literature. The emphasis is upon tendon degeneration rather than inflammation. The clinical picture of pain, swelling, and impaired function is best referred to as Achilles tendinopathy [5]. This terminology may also be applied to the rotator cuff, patellar tendon, and other tendons that have painful overuse

Box 2. Nomenclature in Achilles tendon pain

Clinical
Tendinopathy—pain, swelling, and reduced function
Paratenonopathy—affects paratenon clinically
Panatendinopathy—affects both tendon and paratenon clinically

Histological
Tendinosis—mucoid degeneration and collagen disorganization
Paratenonitis—hyperemia and inflammatory cells; fibrosis and thickening; more common in specimens from younger patients

symptoms [5,7]. The term tendinopathy does not define the underlying pathological processes responsible for the symptoms. In a chronic tendinopathy, there is no inflammatory response and granulation tissue is rarely seen when tissues are examined histologically. For this reason, the term tendinitis is considered inappropriate [3].

The molecular biology of tendinopathy is becoming better understood and is the focus of ongoing research [8]. Laboratory studies of tissue from the insertion of the tendon show necrosis and mucoid degeneration rather than inflammatory infiltration in cases of tendinopathy [9,10].

Local anatomy

To diagnose the cause of posterior heel pain or swelling arising in the region of the Achilles tendon insertion, a thorough understanding of the anatomy is essential (Fig. 1).

Triceps surae

The Achilles tendon is the conjoint tendon of the soleus and the two heads of gastrocnemius. The gastrocnemii originate from the posterior aspect of the femoral condyles and thus span both the knee and the ankle joint. The soleus does not extend above the knee, taking its origin from the posterior aspect of the tibia, fibula, and interosseous membrane [11].

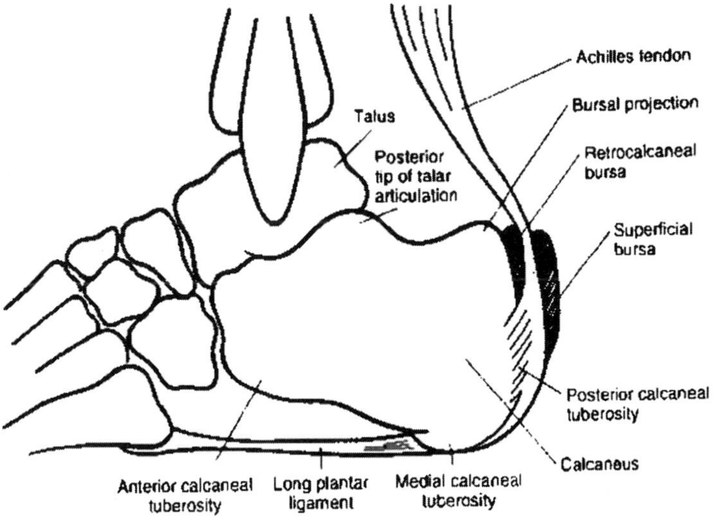

Fig. 1. Posterior heel anatomy. (*From* Stephens MM. Haglund's deformity and retrocalcaneal bursitis. Orthop Clin North Am 1994;25(1):43; with permission.)

This distinction is important when eccentric stretching programs are planned.

The fibers of the conjoint tendon rotate through 90° as they progress distally, such that the medial fibers proximally become the most posterior fibers distally at the insertion [12].

Anatomy at the Achilles insertion

The tendon inserts onto the middle third of the posterior surface of the tuberosity of the os calcis. Like all tendons, insertion into bone is via transitional tissues: tendon, fibrocartilage, mineralized fibrocartilage, and bone. This arrangement is an effective means of force dissipation [13]. That part of the tendon immediately proximal to the insertion is closely related anteriorly to the superior third of the posterior surface of the os calcis. This bone surface may be covered by fibrocartilage [14]. The synovially lined retrocalcaneal bursa lies between tendon and the os calcis at this level. The normal bursa is small, accepting only 1 to 1.5 mL with needle bursography [15]. A subcutaneous bursa lies posterior to the distal Achilles tendon.

Blood supply

The poor blood supply to the noninsertional region of the Achilles tendon is implicated in the pathophysiology of tendinopathy and rupture [16,17]. However, the blood supply to the insertion of the tendon is widely held to be good. The anterior plexus, periosteal vessels, and osseous branches supply this portion of the tendon. Diminished blood flow at the insertion of the tendon has been demonstrated, however, and may play a part in the development of insertional tendinopathy [18].

Bony anatomy

The shape and alignment of the os calcis is relevant to the management of pain or swellings of the posterior heel [19,20]. Distal to the insertion of the Achilles tendon, the os calcis gives attachment to the fascia that runs in continuity with the plantar fascia. An enlarged posterosuperior margin of the calcaneal tuberosity is called a bursal projection (Haglund deformity) and may impinge against the tendon. The impingement may result in retrocalcaneal bursitis or degenerative change in the tendon itself. It may also rub against the heel counter of shoes, producing local swelling and tenderness (pump bumps).

Multiple pathology

Posterior heel pain may be due to degenerative change in the insertional portion of the tendon itself, to enlargement of the retrocalcaneal bursa, or to both. The relevance of an associated Haglund deformity is less clear than previously believed [21]. Pump bumps are usually posterolateral and should not be confused with retrocalcaneal bursitis or insertional tendinopathy. Careful clinical assessment identifies the main pathology and thus guides treatment [22]. The same principle applies to the assessment of patients with noninsertional pain [23].

Insertional tendinopathy

Patients with insertional tendinopathy present with posterior heel pain that is maximal in the central region and at the insertion of the tendon. There is often calcification within the central portion of the Achilles insertion. This calcification can be seen as a spur arising from the middle third of the os calcis on a lateral radiograph (Fig. 2). Laboratory studies in animals show that calcification is intratendinous and forms part of the tendon attachment [24]. Surgical findings in humans, however, demonstrate that the tendon does not gain attachment from this spur [22].

Histology and histochemical studies have shown that an insertional tendinopathy is characterized by mucoid degeneration, necrosis, hemorrhage, and calcification [25].

Retrocalcaneal bursitis

If the posterior heel is swollen and maximally tender away from the midline of the heel, most commonly on the posterolateral aspect, then inflammation within the retrocalcaneal bursa is the likely cause. In many cases,

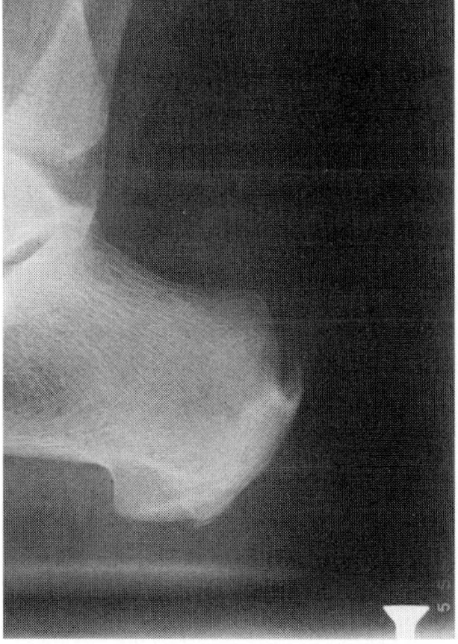

Fig. 2. Lateral radiograph showing calcification seen as a spur arising from the middle third of the os calcis.

this is seen on MRI in conjunction with tendinopathy at the insertion (Fig. 3). The synovium lining the bursa becomes hypertrophic and, although Frey and colleagues [15] found no enlargement of the cavity when contrast was injected, considerable soft tissue swelling and even bony erosion can occur.

Haglund deformity

In the case of a Haglund deformity, a large posterosuperior prominence of the lateral side of the calcaneal tuberosity rubs against poorly fitting shoes. This produces swelling of the subcutaneous (not retrocalcaneal) bursa with a tender, erythematous lump on the heel. In the United States, this has been called a pump bump, emphasizing the association with certain shoes [22].

This condition should be considered as a specific entity, distinct from insertional tendinopathy, although in some cases there is associated enlargement of the retrocalcaneal bursa. Confusion arises because a Haglund deformity may also be seen in up to 60% of patients with insertional Achilles tendinopathy [22]. This does not mean that all patients presenting with pump bumps have insertional tendinopathy [12].

Demographics

Achilles tendinopathy is common, but reliable epidemiological data is not available [26]. An association with athletic training is widely held to be

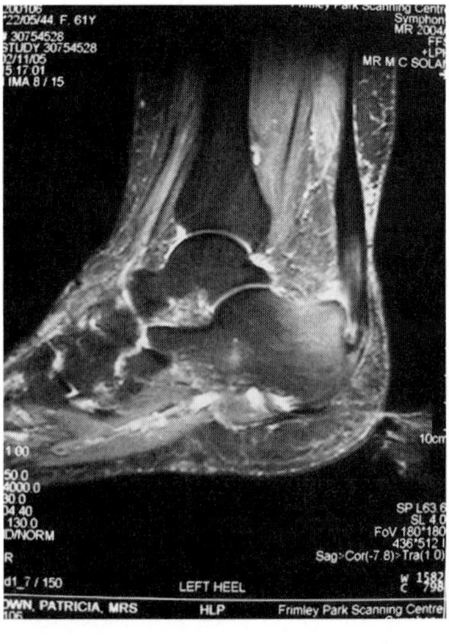

Fig. 3. MRI showing inflammation within the retrocalcaneal bursa.

evidence that overuse is the principal cause [10,27]. Younger athletes have a lower incidence of Achilles pain than older individuals engaged in the same sport [28,29]. Posterior heel pain can, however, affect sedentary individuals as well [12,30]. Schepsis [30] reported that older athletes had a higher prevalence of insertional tendinopathy than did their younger counterparts. Although epidemiological data is limited, existing studies consistently show that noninsertional tendinopathy is four times more prevalent than symptomatic insertional tendonopathy [10,27]. The large study by Paarvola and colleagues [27] from Finland further distinguished between isolated insertional tendinopathy and cases of retrocalcaneal bursitis with insertional tendinopathy. The latter group, with mixed pathology, was much larger, accounting for 20% of all Achilles tendinopathies. Pure insertional tendinopathy made up 5% of the whole cohort.

Measuring Haglund deformity

The presence of a large bursal projection at the posterosuperior margin of the os calcis (Haglund deformity) has been associated with posterior heel pain since its first description in 1928 [31]. Many radiographic measurements have been described in an attempt to define the point at which the posterosuperior margin of the bone becomes excessively prominent [32–36]. Of these measurements, the parallel pitch lines described by Pavlov and colleagues [33] and the superior calcaneal angle described by Philip [34] have been the most enthusiastically adopted by clinicians. Unfortunately, neither method has proven reliable as a guide to treatment. The parallel pitch lines determine the extent to which the bursal projection rises above the rest of the superior surface of the os calcis. Myerson and McGarvey [22] noted that this measurement does not include an assessment of the calcaneal length or pitch. Similarly Stephens [20] reports that, although the superior calcaneal angle of Philip is supposed to be pathological if it exceeds 75°, the measurement does not account for calcaneal pitch.

Lu and colleagues [21] studied these two measurements in a series of weight-bearing radiographs of patients with symptoms of insertional tendinopathy. They compared the findings with those of a control group. There was no statistically significant difference between the two groups in respect of these measurements. Calcification at the Achilles insertion was, however, much more common in the symptomatic group.

Assessment

As with noninsertional Achilles tendinopathy, most patients with insertional symptoms respond to nonoperative treatments [20,22,37–40]. Tailoring the treatment and advice given to the individual patient is essential, and the physician must base treatments on a clear diagnosis as well as on assessment of relevant biomechanics.

History

Careful history-taking determines the relationship of the symptoms to activity, to new training regimens, to poor warm-up technique, or to specific shoes. Atypical features in the history, such as night pain, should prompt investigations to rule out a rare neoplastic cause for the heel pain. Patients with pain arising from the insertion of the tendon, from retrocalcaneal bursitis, or from mixed pathology give a history of pain that is exacerbated by activity. Initially this may be the only symptom. As the condition progresses, the pain becomes constant. Early morning stiffness is typical. Less commonly, swelling is the predominant symptom (Fig. 4).

Examination

Local examination reveals the site of maximal tenderness and the principal cause of the symptoms. Midline tenderness is indicative of insertional tendinopathy, whereas retrocalcaneal bursitis causes maximal tenderness to the lateral (or, less commonly, medial) side of the tendon attachment. Erythema with localized swelling over a superolateral prominence causing a pump bump can also be differentiated by this local examination.

It is important to examine the whole foot and ankle for factors predisposing to the development of posterior heel pain. Increased calcaneal pitch with heel varus renders the bursal projection of the os calcis more prominent and is often a contributory factor in Haglund's disease [20,41]. Excessive heel valgus with a low medial longitudinal arch and forefoot varus causes overpronation of the foot and secondary Achilles tendon injury [42]. Patients with this planovalgus foot posture invariably have adaptive shortening of the gastrocnemius in isolation. This is demonstrated clinically as equinuus deformity at the ankle when tested with the knee extended. Bending the knee relaxes the gastrocnemius and the equinuus deformity is corrected

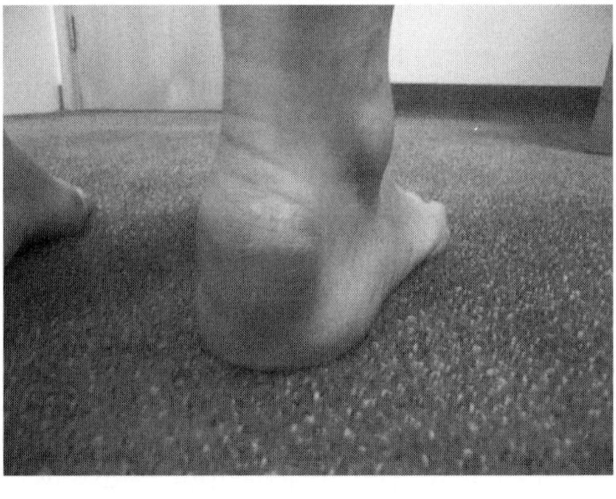

Fig. 4. Clinical photo of a swollen heel.

because the soleus is not tight. This examination technique, described by Silfverskiold [43], must be performed with the forefoot held to reduce the talonavicular joint. If this joint is not reduced, then false-negative findings will occur. This is because the heel escapes into valgus and masks the gastrocnemius contracture by shortening the distance between the knee and the Achilles insertion [44].

Assessment is not complete until the pulses and sensation have been documented. Shoes must be inspected for excessive asymmetrical wear and any orthotic device already in use examined.

If a systemic inflammatory cause is suspected, further physical examination is required and supplemented with appropriate blood tests.

Imaging

Plain radiographs should include a lateral weight-bearing view of the foot and ankle and an axial view of the heel. Any associated postural disorder may mean that further radiographs would be helpful. Anteroposterior weight-bearing views of both feet and an oblique view supplement the weight-bearing lateral film for the assessment of planovalgus deformity. For a foot with cavus deformity, an additional weight-bearing anteroposterior ankle film and mortise view of the ankle are recommended.

Ultrasound scan and MRI can both provide useful information about the tendon and bursae [45]. Neither is required to make the diagnosis, which is made clinically. These modalities are, however, useful for preoperative planning in cases requiring surgical treatment. The principal disadvantage of ultrasound is the absence of a permanent image to which the treating surgeon can usefully refer.

Doppler ultrasound can be used to identify associated neovascularization. Identification of hypervascularity and sclerosant injection treatment is a promising treatment (vide infra).

Treatment

Nonoperative treatment

Orthotics and shoes

Patients with pump bumps respond to education regarding the cause of the symptoms, modification of shoes, and occasionally an orthotic to lift the affected part of the heel away from the upper margin of the heel counter. To avoid recurrence of the problem, the patient must fully understand that he or she must continue to be careful with choice of shoes even after the swelling and tenderness resolve.

Retrocalcaneal bursitis can be managed along similar lines. There may be some benefit from anti-inflammatory medication or gel, but steroid injection should be avoided wherever possible. This is on account of the risk of precipitating rupture of the tendon. If steroid injection is unavoidable, then it should be performed under ultrasound control and the injection placed into the bursa, avoiding the tendon itself. Shoes must be chosen carefully and a heel raise considered. Corrective orthotics for planovalgus deformity can be helpful, but overcorrection is not well tolerated, particularly in runners.

Stretching

Stretching regimens for noninsertional tendinopathy are extremely effective, with 90% of patients responding when the stretches are performed properly [28]. The results in cases of insertional pain are not as good because only one third of patients respond [28]. Stretches are still worth pursuing, particularly where adaptive shortening of the gastrocnemius is pronounced. It is essential that the patient and physiotherapist understand that the knee must be fully extended during the stretch for the gastrocnemius contracture to be improved. Compliance is obviously essential for these stretches to work. If the hamstrings are tight with a large popliteal angle, then stretches for this muscle group should be added to the regimen [46].

"Invasive" nonoperative treatments

Steroid injections should be avoided in disorders of the Achilles tendon. A high proportion of patients presenting with rupture at the insertion of the tendon report prior injection with corticosteroids (Fig. 5) [47]. Where symptoms of retrocalcaneal bursitis predominate, an ultrasound-guided injection

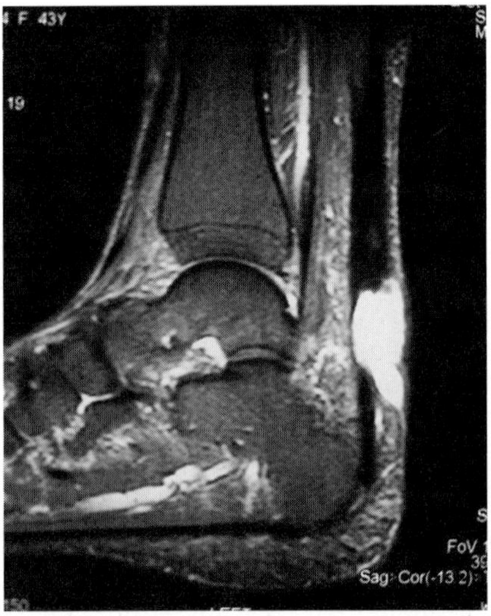

Fig. 5. Rupture after injection of the Achilles tendon.

into the bursa can be considered, as long as both surgeon and patient are aware of the risks.

Sclerosant injection therapy is successful in the treatment of noninsertional tendinopathy [48,49] and has been used for insertional cases in a pilot study. The investigators report good to excellent results in 8 out of 11 cases where neovascularization was demonstrated with Doppler ultrasound [50].

Extracorporeal shock wave lithotripsy is increasingly being evaluated as treatment for chronic soft tissue complaints, including plantar fasciitis, tennis elbow, and rotator cuff injuries. Uptake generally reflects availability of the equipment. There are few reports specific to the treatment of insertional tendinopathy, but their results are promising [51]. Further evidence is needed before extracorporeal shock wave lithotripsy becomes an established treatment option.

Operative treatments

Open procedures

Surgical treatment is reserved for posterior heel pain that has not responded to exhaustive nonoperative treatment. McGarvey and colleagues [47] found that nonoperative treatments were successful in 89% of cases. All investigators involved in the papers reviewed below stress that surgery is only considered for that minority of patients for whom all nonoperative treatments have been tried and have failed to produce sufficient improvement in symptoms.

Comparing the results of different procedures in the literature requires care because it is not always clear whether the reported technique is being used to treat Haglund's disease, retrocalcaneal bursitis, insertional tendinopathy, or a combination of the three.

Haglund's disease alone or in combination with retrocalcaneal bursitis. Haglund's disease that is refractory to nonoperative treatment is rare, and surgical case series therefore have relatively small numbers.

Stephens [20] reported 14 cases and restricts his study to patients without insertional tendinopathy. He recommends excision of the bursal projection through a medial incision, which affords a convenient approach for osteotomy of the posterolateral bony prominence. An additional advantage of this approach is the absence of risk to the sural nerve. This complication is seen when a lateral incision is used [20,22].

Retrocalcaneal bursitis alone. Angermann [52] reviewed patients at an average of 6 years from operation for retrocalcaneal bursitis. The bursa and bursal prominence were resected. Fifty percent of patients were symptom-free and a further 20% were improved. Patients operated on within 1 year of the onset of symptoms fared better, with 92% cured or improved. The result was not affected by the amount of bone removed.

Insertional tendinopathy alone. Maffulli and colleagues [53] treated 21 patients for calcific tendinopathy through a central posterior incision and tendon-splitting approach. The tendon and retrocalcaneal bursa were debrided, but no bone was resected from the bursal projection. At a mean of 4 years after treatment, 11 patients reported excellent results and 5 reported good results. The remaining 5 patients were not sufficiently improved to resume sports.

Johnson and colleagues reviewed 22 patients treated for insertional calcific tendinopathy by tendon detachment, debridement, and reattachment with suture anchors. Average follow-up was 3 years. The American Orthopaedic Foot & Ankle Society (AOFAS) hindfoot score improved from 53 to 89 points with a low rate of complications.

Insertional tendinopathy and/or retrocalcaneal bursitis. Sammarco and Taylor [41] reported excellent results in a larger number of patients where resection of Haglund deformity was performed through a posterior midline Achilles-tendon–splitting approach. In this series, treatment was for insertional tendinopathy and retrocalcaneal bursitis. More recent series use the same tendon-splitting approach and, like Sammarco and Taylor, do not clearly differentiate between Haglund deformity with retrocalcaneal bursitis and tendinopathy of the Achilles insertion [39,47,54].

Sammarco and Taylor's series included 53 sedentary patients with a preponderance of females. Two thirds of the patients failed to improve after an average of more than a year with nonoperative treatments Seventy-five percent of these operated patients were reviewed, with 97% good or excellent results. The Maryland Foot Score was the main outcome measure and improved from 67/100 to 92/100.

Calder and Saxby [54] reported medium-term results of 52 operated heels. Complications were seen only in a patient with psoriatic arthropathy and a bilateral case where both tendons were treated at the same time. Postoperative immobilization was not used in the majority of cases.

McGarvey and colleagues [47] operated upon 22 heels in 21 patients. A central posterior approach was used and the bursal projection resected "as necessary." The satisfaction rate was 82%. Twenty patients resumed normal daily activities within 3 months. Only 13 were able to resume sports activities, however, and 9 patients reported persisting pain. Average follow-up was 33 months.

Wagner and colleagues [39] found good results with debridement alone or in combination with tendon detachment for calcific tendinopathy. They reviewed 61 of a series of 75 patients at an average of 4 years' follow-up. The investigators did not attempt to stratify the results according to the pathology or combination of pathologies. They do note that there was no significant difference in their outcome measures according to whether the tendon was detached and reattached with suture anchors or whether debridement was considered satisfactory without tendon detachment. When the tendon was detached, a proximal V-Y plasty was used in addition.

Retrocalcaneal bursitis versus insertional Achilles tendinopathy with calcific spur. Watson and colleagues [40] recognized that insertional tendinopathy (tendinosis) with calcific spur, retrocalcaneal bursitis, and pump bumps are separate conditions that may coexist. Each condition may cause posterior heel pain as an isolated pathology, or in combination with one or both of the other two pathologies.

They studied the outcome of two groups of patients treated with the same surgical procedure. One group consisted of patients suffering from insertional Achilles tendinopathy with calcific spur only. The second group had signs and symptoms of retrocalcaneal bursitis. This second group included some patients with calcific changes as well, but the clinical diagnosis was retrocalcaneal bursitis. Surgery was performed through a posterolateral incision and the tendon was detached sufficiently to allow proper debridement and resection of the bursal projection. In some, but not all, cases, the tendon was reattached with suture anchors.

There were a number of differences in the recovery times and complication rates between the two groups. Patients with retrocalcaneal bursitis were significantly younger and took 6 months to recover. Those with insertional Achilles tendinopathy and calcific spur required 11 months to recover, were in some cases still restricted in choice of shoe, and suffered a number of complications. There were no complications in the retrocalcaneal bursitis group. The investigators conclude that patients with insertional Achilles tendinopathy and calcific spur have a higher risk of complications and take longer to recover. All of the patients would, however, recommend the treatment to a family member or friend who had the same problem.

Flexor hallucis longus tendon transfer. This reconstructive option is useful in cases of insertional tendon rupture or after extensive debridement. Wong and Ng [55] report good results with all patients able to perform a single-leg heel rise. In this series, all patients were older than 50 years.

Martin and colleagues [56] used this tendon transfer after excision of diseased tendon and reported excellent improvement in pain. Plantarflexion weakness of approximately 30% was noted as the only disadvantage. This did not have significant functional consequences.

Closing wedge osteotomy of the os calcis. A closing wedge osteotomy of the os calcis aims to reduce the posterior prominence of the os calcis [57]. Myerson [22] reports unsatisfactory results, with widening of the heel, a sharp plantar prominence that may require reoperation, and a theoretically diminished lever arm for the Achilles tendon. He recommends the procedure be used in exceptional circumstances, such as, for example, where the os calcis is deformed.

Despite the heterogeneous nature of the literature it is possible to arrive at some generalized conclusions:

- Excision of the bursal projection and debridement of the retrocalcaneal bursa give good results in patients without significant symptoms from the Achilles insertion itself. Some of these patients have calcification at the insertion that is asymptomatic.
- Complete detachment of the Achilles tendon insertion with suture-anchor repair is safe and reliable.
- At least 50% of the attachment can be released without the need for suture-anchor repair and without the need for postoperative cast immobilization. This clinical finding is supported by biomechanical evidence [58].
- There is no consensus regarding the amount of bone that should be removed when the bursal projection is resected. Angermann [52] found no correlation between the amount of bone removed and the outcome. Sella and colleagues [35] recommended that resection be made at an angle of 49° to ensure decompression of the bursa and removal of the calcaneal step.
- Surgical approaches that avoid the risk of sural nerve injury (medial or midline) are preferred to lateral incisions (see Fig. 3).
- Flexor hallucis longus transfer is a useful augmentation.
- Recovery after surgery is not complete for at least 6 months.

Endoscopic debridement of the posterior space

Wound problems after surgery in the region of the Achilles tendon are rare but troublesome. Minimally invasive surgical techniques for debridement to the retrocalcaneal bursa and bursal projection may offer reduced surgical morbidity.

Van Dijk and colleagues [38] reported excellent results in a series of 21 heels (20 patients) treated by endoscopic calcaneoplasty for retrocalcaneal bursitis. There were no complications and a rapid return to normal function. One patient had a fair result whilst the other results were good or excellent. Follow-up was between 2 and 6 years.

Ortmann and McBryde [59] studied a larger group of patients with similar results. Of 30 patients (with 32 operated heels), 28 (30 heels) were followed up at a mean of 3 years. Patients had a clinical diagnosis of retrocalcaneal bursitis. One tendon rupture required repair and 1 patient underwent revision via an open approach. There were no wound complications.

Leitze and colleagues compared results of open versus endoscopic decompression of the retrocalcaneal space. All patients were treated on the basis of the same clinical diagnostic criteria, but this was not a randomized study. Patients with calcification in the tendon insertion were included, unless the spur was greater than 50% of the width of the tendon. Results were good in both groups (total of 33 heels) at 6 to 60 months from surgery. The recovery time was equal in both groups. The endoscopic group had a shorter operative time, fewer wound infections, fewer sensitive scars, and a lower incidence of altered sensation. One patient in the endoscopic group required suture-anchor reattachment of the tendon at the time of debridement.

These reports of endoscopic treatment show that results are at least as good as those after open treatment. Recommendations can be based upon these reports:

- Intraoperative fluoroscopy is advisable to ensure that the extent of bony resection meets the preoperative plan.
- The risk of conversion to open debridement or of tendon detachment is small, but patients should be warned that either of these eventualities would mean a larger scar and the need for postoperative cast protection.
- Operating theater staff should be asked to ensure that suture anchors are available.
- Patients must be counseled that "key-hole" surgery does not always equate to rapid recovery.

Authors' preferred treatment

The authors believe that an accurate assessment of the source of pain guides treatment. Nonoperative treatment is preferred initially. Steroid injection is avoided wherever possible and, if performed, ultrasound guidance is used. The patient is counseled regarding the risk of rupture. For recalcitrant cases, surgery has good results (Box 3). If an isolated gastrocnemius contracture cannot be corrected by physiotherapy, a gastrocnemius

Box 3. Treatment Algorithm

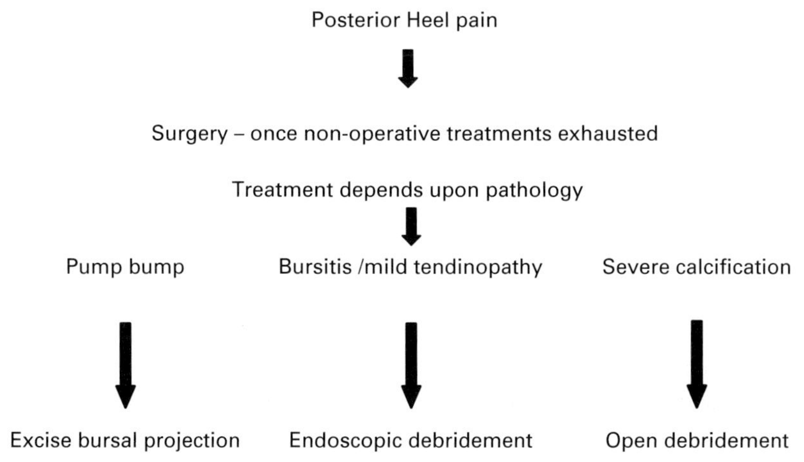

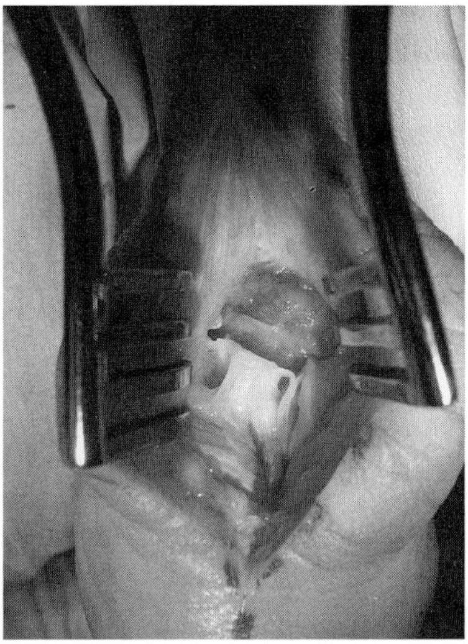

Fig. 6. Posterior midline approach.

release is considered. As with eccentric physiotherapy stretches, the results are less reliable than for the treatment of noninsertional tendinopathy. Isolated Haglund deformity is treated by reduction of the bursal projection. Retrocalcaneal bursitis with mild insertional tendinopathy is debrided endoscopically. Where the calcific spur is large, an open debridement is preferred through a posterior midline incision and tendon-splitting approach (Fig. 6). If less than half the insertion is detached, postoperative cast immobilization is not routinely employed. In the authors' experience, complete detachment of the tendon is not necessary. If the patient presents with rupture at the insertion, the authors recommend augmentation with transfer of flexor hallucis longus. If the distal stump is suitable, then the flexor hallucis longus is split and a side-to-side tenodesis used. If the distal stump is too diseased, a short harvest, calcaneal tunnel, and interference screw fixation is the preferred technique.

References

[1] Clain MR, Baxter DE. Achilles tendinitis. Foot Ankle 1992;13(8):482–7.

[2] Daniels TR. Osteochondroses of the foot. In: Myerson MS, editor. Foot and ankle disorders., vol. 2. 1st edition. Philadelphia: WB Saunders; 2000. p. 797–8.

[3] Khan KM, Cook JL, Kannus P, et al. Time to abandon the "tendinitis" myth. BMJ 2002; 324(7338):626–7.

[4] Krishna Sayana M, Maffulli N. Insertional Achilles tendinopathy. Foot Ankle Clin 2005; 10(2):309–20.

[5] Maffulli N, Khan KM, Puddu G. Overuse tendon conditions: time to change a confusing terminology. Arthroscopy 1998;14(8):840–3.

[6] Sharma P, Maffulli N. Understanding and managing achilles tendinopathy. Br J Hosp Med (Lond) 2006;67(2):64–7.
[7] Maffulli N, Cook JL, Khan KM. Re: Recalcitrant patellar tendinosis in elite athletes: surgical treatment in conjunction with aggressive postoperative rehabilitation. Am J Sports Med 2006;34(8):1364, [author reply: 1364–5].
[8] Magra M, Maffulli N. Molecular events in tendinopathy: a role for metalloproteases. Foot Ankle Clin 2005;10(2):267–77.
[9] Kvist M. Achilles tendon injuries in athletes. Sports Med 1994;18(3):173–201.
[10] Astrom M, Rausing A. Chronic Achilles tendinopathy. A survey of surgical and histopathologic findings. Clin Orthop Relat Res 1995;316:151–64.
[11] O'Brien M. The anatomy of the Achilles tendon. Foot Ankle Clin 2005;10(2):225–38.
[12] Mandelbaum B. Disorders of the Achilles tendon and the retrocalcaneal region. In: Myerson MS, editor. Foot and Ankle Disorders, vol. 2. 1st edition. Philadelphia: WB Saunders; 2000. p. 1367–98.
[13] Benjamin M, Evans EJ, Copp L. The histology of tendon attachments to bone in man. J Anat 1986;149:89–100.
[14] Rufai A, Ralphs JR, Benjamin M. Ultrastructure of fibrocartilages at the insertion of the rat Achilles tendon. J Anat 1996;189(Pt 1):185–91.
[15] Frey C, Rosenberg Z, Shereff MJ, et al. The retrocalcaneal bursa: anatomy and bursography. Foot Ankle 1992;13(4):203–7.
[16] Carr AJ, Norris SH. The blood supply of the calcaneal tendon. J Bone Joint Surg Br 1989; 71(1):100–1.
[17] Lagergren C, Lindholm A. Vascular distribution in the Achilles tendon: an angiographic and microangiographic study. Acta Chir Scand 1959;116(5–6):491–5.
[18] Schmidt-Rohlfing B, Graf J, Schneider U, et al. The blood supply of the Achilles tendon. Int Orthop 1992;16(1):29–31.
[19] Keener BJ, Sizensky JA. The anatomy of the calcaneus and surrounding structures. Foot Ankle Clin 2005;10(3):413–24.
[20] Stephens MM. Haglund's deformity and retrocalcaneal bursitis. Orthop Clin North Am 1994;25(1):41–6.
[21] Lu CC, Cheng YM, Fu YC, et al. Angle analysis of Haglund syndrome and its relationship with osseous variations and achilles tendon calcification. Foot Ankle Int 2007;28(2):181–5.
[22] Myerson MS, McGarvey W. Disorders of the Achilles tendon insertion and Achilles tendinitis. Instr Course Lect 1999;48:211–8.
[23] Maffulli N, Kenward MG, Testa V, et al. Clinical diagnosis of Achilles tendinopathy with tendinosis. Clin J Sport Med 2003;13(1):11–5.
[24] Benjamin M, Rufai A, Ralphs JR. The mechanism of formation of bony spurs (enthesophytes) in the achilles tendon. Arthritis Rheum 2000;43(3):576–83.
[25] Merkel KH, Hess H, Kunz M. Insertion tendopathy in athletes. A light microscopic, histochemical and electron microscopic examination. Pathol Res Pract 1982;173(3):303–9.
[26] Maffulli N, Wong J, Almekinders LC. Types and epidemiology of tendinopathy. Clin Sports Med 2003;22(4):675–92.
[27] Paavola M, Orava S, Leppilahti J, et al. Chronic Achilles tendon overuse injury: complications after surgical treatment. An analysis of 432 consecutive patients. Am J Sports Med 2000;28(1):77–82.
[28] Fahlstrom M, Jonsson P, Lorentzon R, et al. Chronic Achilles tendon pain treated with eccentric calf-muscle training. Knee Surg Sports Traumatol Arthrosc 2003;11(5):327–33.
[29] Fahlstrom M, Lorentzon R, Alfredson H. Painful conditions in the Achilles tendon region: a common problem in middle-aged competitive badminton players. Knee Surg Sports Traumatol Arthrosc 2002;10(1):57–60.
[30] Schepsis AA, Jones H, Haas AL. Achilles tendon disorders in athletes. Am J Sports Med 2002;30(2):287–305.
[31] Haglund P. Beitrag Zur Klinik der Achillessehne. Aschr Orthop Chir 1928;49:49–58.

[32] Chauveaux D, Liet P, Le Huec JC, et al. A new radiologic measurement for the diagnosis of Haglund's deformity. Surg Radiol Anat 1991;13(1):39–44.

[33] Pavlov H, Heneghan MA, Hersh A, et al. The Haglund syndrome: initial and differential diagnosis. Radiology 1982;144(1):83–8.

[34] Philip AFJ. Abnormality of the calcaneus as a cause of painful heel: its diagnosis and operative treatment. Br J Surg 1945;32:494–8.

[35] Sella EJ, Caminear DS, McLarney EA. Haglund's syndrome. J Foot Ankle Surg 1998;37(2): 110–4, [discussion: 173].

[36] Steffensen JC, Evensen A. Bursitis retrocalcanea achilli. Acta Orthop Scand 1958;27(3): 229–36.

[37] Clement DB, Taunton JE, Smart GW. Achilles tendinitis and peritendinitis: etiology and treatment. Am J Sports Med 1984;12(3):179–84.

[38] van Dijk CN, van Dyk GE, Scholten PE, et al. Endoscopic calcaneoplasty. Am J Sports Med 2001;29(2):185–9.

[39] Wagner E, Gould JS, Kneidel M, et al. Technique and results of Achilles tendon detachment and reconstruction for insertional Achilles tendinosis. Foot Ankle Int 2006;27(9):677–84.

[40] Watson AD, Anderson RB, Davis WH. Comparison of results of retrocalcaneal decompression for retrocalcaneal bursitis and insertional achilles tendinosis with calcific spur. Foot Ankle Int 2000;21(8):638–42.

[41] Sammarco GJ, Taylor AL. Operative management of Haglund's deformity in the nonathlete: a retrospective study. Foot Ankle Int 1998;19(11):724–9.

[42] James SL, Bates BT, Osternig LR. Injuries to runners. Am J Sports Med 1978;6(2):40–50.

[43] Silfverskiold N. Uber die subkutane totale Achillessehnenruptur and deren Behandlung. Acta Chir Scand 1941;84:393.

[44] DiGiovanni CW, Kuo R, Tejwani N, et al. Isolated gastrocnemius tightness. J Bone Joint Surg Am 2002;84-A(6):962–70.

[45] Bleakney RR, White LM. Imaging of the Achilles tendon. Foot Ankle Clin 2005;10(2): 239–54.

[46] Harty J, Soffe K, O'Toole G, et al. The role of hamstring tightness in plantar fasciitis. Foot Ankle Int 2005;26(12):1089–92.

[47] McGarvey WC, Palumbo RC, Baxter DE, et al. Insertional Achilles tendinosis: surgical treatment through a central tendon splitting approach. Foot Ankle Int 2002;23(1):19–25.

[48] Ohberg L, Alfredson H. Ultrasound guided sclerosis of neovessels in painful chronic Achilles tendinosis: pilot study of a new treatment. Br J Sports Med 2002;36(3):173–5, [discussion: 176–7].

[49] Alfredson H, Ohberg L. Sclerosing injections to areas of neo-vascularisation reduce pain in chronic Achilles tendinopathy: a double-blind randomised controlled trial. Knee Surg Sports Traumatol Arthrosc 2005;13(4):338–44.

[50] Ohberg L, Alfredson H. Sclerosing therapy in chronic Achilles tendon insertional pain—results of a pilot study. Knee Surg Sports Traumatol Arthrosc 2003;11(5):339–43.

[51] Furia JP. High-energy extracorporeal shock wave therapy as a treatment for insertional Achilles tendinopathy. Am J Sports Med 2006;34(5):733–40.

[52] Angermann P. Chronic retrocalcaneal bursitis treated by resection of the calcaneus. Foot Ankle 1990;10(5):285–7.

[53] Maffulli N, Testa V, Capasso G, et al. Calcific insertional Achilles tendinopathy: reattachment with bone anchors. Am J Sports Med 2004;32(1):174–82.

[54] Calder JD, Saxby TS. Surgical treatment of insertional Achilles tendinosis. Foot Ankle Int 2003;24(2):119–21.

[55] Wong MW, Ng VW. Modified flexor hallucis longus transfer for Achilles insertional rupture in elderly patients. Clin Orthop Relat Res 2005;431:201–6.

[56] Martin RL, Manning CM, Carcia CR, et al. An outcome study of chronic Achilles tendinosis after excision of the Achilles tendon and flexor hallucis longus tendon transfer. Foot Ankle Int 2005;26(9):691–7.

[57] Keck SW, Kelly PJ. Bursitis of the posterior part of the heel; evaluation of surgical treatment of eighteen patients. J Bone Joint Surg Am 1965;47:267–73.
[58] Kolodziej P, Glisson RR, Nunley JA. Risk of avulsion of the Achilles tendon after partial excision for treatment of insertional tendonitis and Haglund's deformity: a biomechanical study. Foot Ankle Int 1999;20(7):433–7.
[59] Ortmann FW, McBryde AM. Endoscopic bony and soft-tissue decompression of the retrocalcaneal space for the treatment of Haglund deformity and retrocalcaneal bursitis. Foot Ankle Int 2007;28(2):149–53.

ELSEVIER
SAUNDERS

Foot Ankle Clin N Am
12 (2007) 617–641

FOOT AND
ANKLE CLINICS

Noninsertional Achilles Tendinopathy

Michael S. Hennessy, BSc, FRCSEd (Tr&Orth)[a,*], Andrew P. Molloy, FRCS (Tr&Orth)[b], Simon W. Sturdee, FRCS (Tr&Orth)[a]

[a] *Wirral Hospitals NHS Trust, Upton, Wirral, CH49 5PE, UK*
[b] *Royal Liverpool University Hospital, Liverpool, UK*

> Achilles was the mightiest of the Greeks to fight in the Trojan War. In an effort to make him immortal, his mother Thetis held the young Achilles by the heel and dipped him into the River Styx; everything the sacred waters touched became invulnerable. His heel remained dry and was thus unprotected. Achilles was wounded in his heel by an arrow and died from his wound [1].

Thus, since the ancients, has the Achilles tendon been problematic and is now the downfall of many a weekend warrior in the twenty-first century. For the most part, treatment has been variable and often contradictory, with similar degrees of success with seemingly different approaches being reported from different countries and different clinics within the same country. Even the terminology has been confusing, with several names being used for apparently the same condition: tendonitis, tendinitis, paratenonitis, tendovaginitis, tenosynovitis, achillodynia, and others [2]. For clarity, the clinical syndrome of (activity-related) pain and swelling of the body of the Achilles tendon with impaired performance is referred to in this article as noninsertional Achilles tendinopathy [3,4]. This is a clinical diagnosis and may include the histopathological diagnoses of peritendinitis and tendinosis [5], the latter seen in surgical specimens in which there is a poor and disordered healing response within the damaged tendon and an absence of the "normal" inflammatory cell infiltrate and biochemical mediators (eg, prostaglandin E2) [6]. Hence the suffix -opathy, rather than -itis, is correct.

Much clinical and basic scientific research has been done and continues to be done. Yet, the management of this condition still tends to be empirical, based on experience, philosophy, and art, rather than evidence. The busy

* Corresponding author.
E-mail address: mchenno@btinternet.com (M.S. Hennessy).

doi:10.1016/j.fcl.2007.07.006
foot.theclinics.com

clinician is faced with an overwhelming volume of literature discussing etiology, pathology, and treatment with few clear-cut answers. Thankfully, because of the work of many, but most notably Maffulli and colleagues [7,8], logic and science are being applied to bring a semblance of order to the mass of information available about this increasingly common condition.

The authors attempt in this article to distill the currently available information into something user-friendly to the foot and ankle surgeon.

Epidemiology and classification

Achilles tendinopathy is common in the general population and is usually, but not exclusively, seen as a consequence of participation in sports. It tends to be an overuse problem and is the "runner's disease" with an annual incidence of 7% to 9% in top level runners [9,10] and prevalence in runners of an estimated 11%, but any strenuous activity involving running and jumping can be implicated. As recreational, competitive, and professional sports increase among the general population, so does the incidence of sports-related injuries, Achilles tendinopathy being one of the most common presentations [11]. In studies of conditions affecting the Achilles tendon, 66% are noninsertional Achilles tendinopathy [12,13]. Most patients tend to be male, running is the main sport (53%), and the affected population tends to be older athletes (as opposed to teenage and child athletes).

Attempts to classify the condition have been somewhat arbitrary with symptoms over 6 weeks' duration being termed as "chronic" [14]. Otherwise classification has been based upon histological findings with various types of degeneration—hypoxic, hyaline, mucoid, fibrinoid, fatty, and calcific—all found within surgical specimens.

Anatomy

The gastrocnemius and soleus muscles in the calf merge to form the Achilles tendon, which is the strongest and largest tendon in the body. The muscles that form the Achilles tendon originate in the posterior-superior compartment of the calf. Their main action is to plantarflex the ankle. The medial and lateral heads of the gastrocnemius with the plantaris cross the knee joint so that when the knee is extended and the ankle dorsiflexed the muscle is stretched. The gastrocnemius muscle fibers are mostly fast-twitch fibers and flex the foot on the ankle and also flex the knee, having the action of propelling the body in a forward direction in gait. The soleus muscle is a postural muscle and its fibers are mostly slow-twitch type I fibers. The soleus muscle also acts as a peripheral vascular pump.

The soleus muscle is a broad, flat multipennate muscle and is wider than the gastrocnemius. The muscle fibers of the soleus muscle extend more distally than those of the gastrocnemius. The soleus muscle lies under the gastrocnemius muscle, originates from the posterior surface of the upper tibia and fibula and from the interposed tendinous arch. The gastrocnemius muscle is the most superficial muscle in the calf and is fusiform, forming the inferior boundary of the popliteal fossa. The muscle has two heads that originate from the posterior aspect of the femoral condyles. The medial head is larger than the lateral head and extends more distally in the calf. The deep surface of the gastrocnemius that lies on the soleus muscle is tendinous. The two muscle bellies of gastrocnemius extend to the middle of the calf and form a tendinous raphe that becomes continuous with the aponeurosis on the deep surface of the muscle. This merges with the tendon of soleus to form a conjoined tendon, the Achilles tendon.

The tendon proximally is rounded and is relatively flat distally. Approximately 12 to 15 cm proximal to its insertion, rotation of the tendon begins and this becomes more marked in the distal 5 to 6 cm. The tendon spirals approximately 90° with the medial fibers rotating posteriorly. This twisting produces stress within the tendon. This stress has been shown to be greatest 2 to 5 cm above the calcaneal insertion, which is the common site for tendinopathy and rupture [15,16]. This site is also an area of poor vascularity (vide infra).

The tendon inserts on the posterior surface of the calcaneus distal to the posterior-superior calcaneal tuberosity. The insertion becomes broad distally and has a deltoid-type attachment, which ranges from 1.2 to 2.5 cm [17]. The retrocalcaneal bursa lies deep and just proximal to the insertion of the Achilles tendon and lies between the tuberosity on the posterior surface of the calcaneus and the tendon.

The Achilles tendon receives its blood supply from intrinsic and extrinsic systems: intrinsic at the myotendinous and osteotendinous junctions and extrinsic via the paratenon. Doppler studies have demonstrated a zone of relative hypovascularity 2 to 7 cm proximal to the tendon insertion [18–20], the same region involved in noninsertional tendinopathy. Nerve fibers similarly form a rich plexus in the paratenon and likewise penetrate the epitenon with vascular counterparts, although most terminate as nerve endings on the tendon surface.

Tendon structure

A healthy tendon is white with a fibroelastic texture. Collagen (about 95% is type I collagen and 5% is type III and IV) and elastin fibers are embedded in an extracellular matrix of proteoglycan and water. The cellular component (90%–95%) of tendon is made up of tenoblasts and mature tenocytes, the remaining cells being chondrocytes at bone attachments, synovial cells of tendon sheaths, and vascular cells [21]. These cells lie in and produce the extracellular matrix consisting of collagen type 1 (65%–80% dry mass) and elastin (2%). The collagen is arranged in a hierarchical structure in which triple helix polypeptide chains unite into fibrils, which are grouped into fibers, arranged into fascicles, which grouped together form the tendon itself.

Tendons through their ultrastructure exhibit viscoelastic and other biomechanical properties. At rest, the collagen fibers adopt a "crimped" configuration. Application of increasing stress causes a stretch or strain. A strain of up to 2% stretches out the crimped pattern. Beyond this, tendons deform in a linear fashion on a stress/strain curve because of intermolecular sliding of the collagen. Strains of up to 4% behave in an elastic fashion, returning to original shape once the deforming force (stress) has been removed. Strains above 8% to 10%, however, cause microscopic failure due to "molecular slippage" (Fig. 1). What is important in tendon failure is not only the amount of force applied but also the rate and direction of the applied force.

Etiology

The Achilles tendon is subjected to the largest loads of any tendon in the body. Tensile loads of up to 10 times body weight during running, jumping, hopping, and skipping have been shown [22–25]. Achilles tendinopathy, though it can be seen in both athletic and nonathletic individuals and though its cause remains unclear, is certainly associated with overuse and repetitive loading. Pathogenesis is largely felt to be multifactorial, with mechanical, vascular, and neural components in combination.

The nature and cause of pain in tendinopathy remain unclear. Classically thought to be as a consequence of inflammation, chronically painful Achilles tendons have shown no evidence of inflammation and, by the same measure, intratendinous lesions can be seen on MRI without pain as a symptom. Current theories propose increased levels of substance P and glutamate

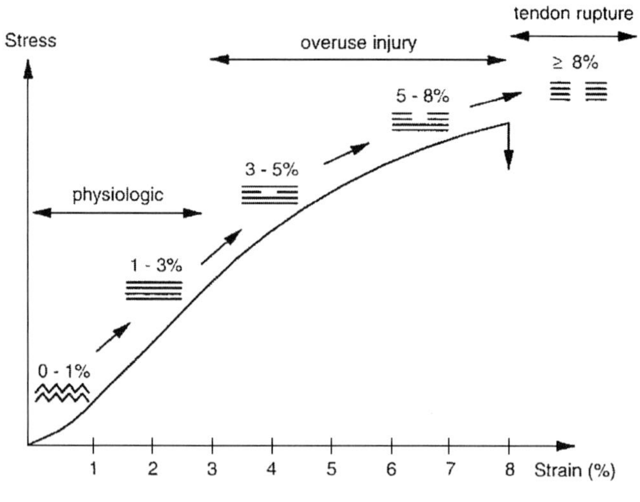

Fig. 1. Development of chronic tendon disorders. (*From* Jarvinen TAH, Kannus P, Maffulli N, et al. Achilles tendon disorders: etiology and epidemiology. Foot Ankle Clin 2005;10: 260; with permission.)

(both neurotransmitters) found in degenerate tendons as possible culprits [6,26,27]. Degeneration and collagen breakdown may also be factors.

The many factors that have been associated with causing Achilles tendinopathy can be subdivided into intrinsic and extrinsic factors and can occur alone or in combination. A list of these factors can be seen in tables described by Kannus [28] and Järvinen and colleagues [29].

Poor vascularity, dysfunction of the gastrocnemius-soleus, advanced age, male gender, above average body weight and height, deformity (eg, pes cavus), and lateral instability of the ankle are considered common intrinsic factors. Others are shown in Box 1.

Excessive movement of the hindfoot in the frontal plane, especially at lateral heel strike with excessive compensatory "hyper-" or "overpronation" is thought to cause a "whipping action" on the Achilles tendon, predisposing to tendinopathy (see Box 1) [12]. This particular and reasonable premise has also led to the current explosion of functional foot orthoses being provided on the high street for hiking and walking boots as well as for running shoes with sales promoted by many theories, not all of which are well founded.

Box 1. Intrinsic factors shown to predispose to Achilles tendinopathy

General factors
Male gender
Age >50
Above average weight
Constitution: weak or strong
Blood group
HLA type
Predisposing diseases
Blood supply (ischemia, hypoxia, hyperthermia)

Local anatomic factors in the lower limb
Malalignments
- Foot hyper- or hypopronation
- Forefoot varus or valgus
- Hindfoot varus or valgus
- Pes planus or cavus

Leg-length discrepancy
Muscle weakness and imbalance
Decreased flexibility
Joint laxity

From Jarvinen TAH, Kannus P, Maffulli N, et al. Achilles tendon disorders: etiology and epidemiology. Foot Ankle Clin 2005;10:260; with permission.

Histopathological examination of tendon specimens from patients with the clinical syndrome of activity-related swelling and pain in the midsubstance of the Achilles tendon show noninflammatory collagen degeneration and a disordered healing response with a distinct absence of the normal inflammatory response. What has also been seen in tendinopathy are imbalances in the levels of matrix metalloproteases (MMPs), a family of proteolyic enzymes involved in the remodelling the extracellular matrix, and their antagonists, the tissue inhibitors of MMPs (TIMPs). Tendon damage is seen to up- and down-regulate members of these enzyme families in such a way that normal remodelling and maintenance of tendons are affected [30]. While related research is in its infancy, this finding may indicate a future direction for treatment.

A vascular theory of causes is based on the fact that tendons are metabolically active and any compromise to the vascular supply may lead to degeneration, as repair of microtrauma described previously will not occur. This vascular compromise may be worse during exercise [31]. A zone of hypovascularity 2 to 6 cm proximal to the tendon insertion corresponds with the site of pathology in tendinopathy [18–20,32–34]. Many treatments use this theory by attempting to stimulate neovascularization.

Of the extrinsic factors responsible for Achilles tendinopathy, training errors, overtraining, poor technique, and fatigue undoubtedly play a major part, even though randomized studies of interventions in these are lacking. Excess loading due to whatever reason—overzealous training or unaccustomed physical exercise, for example—is probably the main stimulus for degeneration or inflammation, the tendon's response to repetitive overload. Failure to repair damage leads to weakness and rupture. Repetitive microtrauma may not allow sufficient time for repair. This would be logical. Indeed, certain chemicals—fluorquinolone antibiotics in particular [35,36]—inhibit tenocyte metabolism and have been implicated in Achilles tendinopathy.

While inflammatory exudate is seen to be lacking in specimens from chronic tendon degeneration in the acute phase, crepitus is very often elicited clinically. This elicitation of crepitus is due to fibrinous exudate in the paratenon, which can lead to peritendinous adhesions and possibly tendinosis, the basis for most of the open surgical treatments that involve decompression and debridement of the paratenon in particular. However, these two conditions—peritendinopathy and tendinosis—can coexist or occur in isolation and as yet no temporal relationship has been convincingly demonstrated. Exercise-induced hyperthermia and free radical production have also been implicated in tendinopathy (Box 2) [37].

Tendon healing

Tendons, like most other tissues, heal in separate but overlapping phases. The first phase is the inflammatory phase, when cellular debris is removed by macrophages and there is the secretion of cytokines and chemotactic

Box 2. Extrinsic factors related to Achilles tendinopathy in sports

General factors

Therapeutic agents
- Corticosteroids (local and systemic)

Fluorquinolone
- Antibiotics
- Weight-lowering drugs

Drugs
- Anabolic steroids

Drugs/narcotics
- Cannabis
- Heroin
- Cocaine

Sports-related factors

Excessive loads on the lower extremities
- Speed of movement
- Type of movement
- Number of repetitions
- Footwear, sportswear
- Training surface

Training errors
- Overdistance
- Fast progression
- High intensity
- Fatigue
- Poor technique

Environmental conditions
- Heat or cold
- Humidity
- Altitude
- Wind

Poor equipment

From Jarvinen TAH, Kannus P, Maffulli N, et al. Achilles tendon disorders: etiology and epidemiology. Foot Ankle Clin 2005;10:260; with permission.

agents from neutrophils in particular, stimulating angiogenesis, vascular permeability, and tenocyte proliferation. The second phase is the proliferative phase, with production of type 3 collagen and changes in the composition of the extracellular matrix. The final, remodeling phase, then occurs at about 6 weeks' postinjury when type 1 collagen synthesis increases, cellular to fibrous changes occur, and scar-like repair tissue appears. This pattern of healing is determined by the tendon and its constituent cells and may be influenced by the type of trauma and location of insult. The exact mechanisms involved remain elusive but certainly implicate MMPs, nitric oxide, and tenocyte origin and phenotypic expression.

Most treatment strategies aim to stimulate, modify, or inhibit various stages of the processes above.

Clinical presentation

As with all conditions, a detailed clinical history, including time of onset, duration of symptoms, previous episodes, exacerbating and relieving factors, medications, and previous attempted therapies, provide valuable information in determining the approach in the individual patient.

Examination should elicit the site or sites of tenderness, areas of warmth, and localized deformity. A clinical examination of lower limbs as a whole may provide clues as to etiology. Examples of such clues are limb-length discrepancy, ankle instability, cavovarus deformity, generalized laxity, or decreased flexibility.

The common pattern of presentation includes morning stiffness and a gradual onset of pain during activity. In severe cases, pain occurs at rest.

Imaging

Plain radiography

The authors do not routinely recommend plain radiographs in every patient with Achilles tendinopathy, although valuable information may be obtained in the less clear-cut cases. Plain radiographs show erosions and the presence of abnormal calcification or ossification around the hindfoot.

Ulrasound

Ultrasound is a quick, safe, relatively available, and noninvasive imaging modality and allows easy contralateral comparison. However, ultrasound is certainly very operator-dependant and gives limited information. Ultrasonic evaluation of the tendon should be performed in transverse and longitudinal planes [38]. The normal tendon gives an echogenic pattern of parallel lines. The bursae at the tendon insertion on to the calcaneus can also be well visualized. On transverse imaging, the tendon has an anteroposterior thickness of 4 to 6 mm, with 6 mm the upper limit of normal. Thus, the thickening apparent in tendinopathy is easily determined and, because most cases tend to be unilateral, comparison with the "normal" side can be made. In patients with clinical tendinopathy, focal "hypoechoic" areas correspond to areas of degeneration but can be reported as "spontaneous" or "partial ruptures" and thus can be misleading to the inexperienced clinician. True partial tears are rarely seen at surgery.

MRI

MRI is the current gold standard for imaging the Achilles tendon. Excellent soft tissue visualization and multiplanar imaging provide excellent assessment of the tendon. Tendinopathy manifests as fusiform thickening and areas of increased signal, particularly on the T-2–weighted sequences representing collagen fiber degeneration. MRI has also, unlike ultrasound, been seen to correlate with 12-month clinical outcomes (Fig. 2) [39].

Treatment

For many years, management of tendinopathy of the body of the Achilles tendon was based on anecdotal evidence with little understanding of the causes and pathogenesis of the condition. Thus, most older studies were retrospective in nature with no element of randomization and contained fairly heterogeneous groups. Treatment was aimed at symptom relief and as usual fell into either operative or nonoperative/conservative groups. Most clinicians recommended operative intervention only after 3 to 6 months of unsuccessful conservative management. However, nonoperative treatment has been seen to fail in a third of patients in one of the few long-term follow-up studies [40,41]. In spite of this, the authors still recommend initial nonoperative management in early phases of tendinopathy because operative treatments also have variable outcomes ranging from 75% to 100%

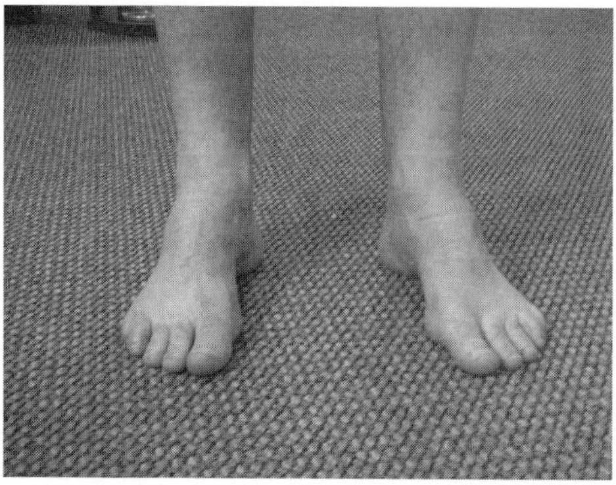

Fig. 2. Intrinsic factors: bilateral cavovarus attitude of feet in patient who has Achilles tendinopathy.

success rates based on retrospective studies with subjective rather than objective outcomes [7,13,24,41–53].

Nonoperative treatments

Traditional nonoperative modalities have had little scientific basis and have included such strategies as rest (either modified or complete), orthoses, pharmacological agents (including nonsteroidal anti-inflammatory drugs (NSAIDS) and corticosteroid injections), and various physical therapies and modalities. Results of traditional methods have had varying success rates, ranging from 50% to 81% [2,40,41]. However, this course of management should be seen as a combination of strategies aimed at symptom control and patient education.

Training errors should be addressed, with the avoidance of repetitive, monotonous training, such as running alone, and the introduction of cross-training methods. Likewise, running too great a distance or running at too great an intensity or too rapidly should be avoided. Limb malalignment and flexibility should also be addressed with the help of physiotherapy and orthotics.

Pharmacological agents

Nonsteroidal anti-inflammatory drugs. The use of NSAIDS in both acute and chronic Achilles tendinopathies is widespread, although there is little scientific evidence for their use. While they certainly help in pain control, the mechanism of action is elusive.

There is debate in acute tendinopathies about whether blockade of the inflammatory response is beneficial or not [54]. In animal models, cyclooxygenase-2 inhibitors were found to have inhibited tendon cell migration and proliferation, although expression of collagen types I and III remained unchanged [55]. In another rat model, cyclooygenase-1 and -2 inhibitors were found to have no detrimental effect on tendon tensile strength and the only benefit demonstrated was a reduction in cross-sectional area of the model tendon [56,57]. The investigators hypothesized that this would only be of benefit where thickening of a healing tendon could be problematical. In the authors' experience, this symptom is not usually the patient's primary complaint. Diclofenac has been shown in rat Achilles tendon to reduce edema and accumulation of neutrophils and $CD1^{+}$ macrophages in the area around the paratenon. However, these effects were not found in the central core of the tendon. There was no functional or biochemical benefit demonstrated [58].

As there is little or no inflammatory cell infiltrate demonstrated in the chronic setting [59,60], the benefit of NSAIDS in chronic tendinopathy is questionable. Further doubts about NSAIDs have been raised clinically by a double-blind placebo-controlled study that found piroxicam not to be of significant benefit. Meanwhile, a Cochrane review [61] stated that there was at best weak clinical evidence for the use of NSAIDs in Achilles tendinopathies.

Corticosteroid injections. Corticosteroid injections have also historically been used in the treatment of acute Achilles tendinopathy, but the popularity of such injections is waning. The adverse risks of intratendinous injections are well documented. Partial ruptures can be found following these injections, although the cause of these ruptures is uncertain. According to one hypothesis, the ruptures stem directly from corticosteroid injections. According to another hypothesis, the ruptures are the result of inherent tendon abnormalities that morphologically alter the tendon, leading to excessive strain. According to a third hypothesis, the ruptures occur because pain has been masked so much that excessive strain is not detected [45,62–64]. Meta-analysis of the effects of corticosteroid injections has shown little benefit and there is insufficient evidence to accurately predict the exact rupture rate [65]. However, intratendinous injection should always be avoided because of the risk of direct pressure effects causing serious hypoxic injury. Other risks, such as fat atrophy and skin hyperpigmentation or hypopigmentation, are also well known. The safety of using corticosteroid injections can be enhanced with the use of imaging as a guide for entering only the peritendinous space. However, the results of this technique—53% of patients stated that their condition was unchanged and 7% stated that they were worse off—are disappointing [66].

Topical glyceryl trinitrate. A prospective double-blind randomized study involving 65 patients compared the continuous application of topical glyceryl trinitrate (GTN) with rehabilitation alone [67]. At 6 months, 78% of the patients in the GTN group were asymptomatic compared with 49% in the placebo group, a significant difference. The rationale behind this treatment is that nitric oxide in animal models seems to stimulate collagen synthesis in fibroblasts.

Orthotics

Orthotics are widely used in conservative management, with heel pads being the most commonly prescribed. These are classically up to 12 to 15 mm in height [24]. There is little evidence to support their use with one of the few scientifically robust studies (observer-blinded, randomized, and prospective) by Lowdon and colleagues [68] showing no benefit at 10 days' and 2 months' follow-up. In the overly pronated hindfoot, biomechanical principles suggest that increased stress might be placed on the medial part of the Achilles tendon as the hindfoot further pronates during the stance phase of gait. However, no controlled scientific evidence supports that a correction to an overly pronated hindfoot is beneficial, although anecdotal evidence and certainly patient peer pressure seems to drive this treatment. Other devices have been seen to be helpful both in the acute and chronic stages of treatment. Such devices include the AchilloTrain brace (Bauerfeind AG, Zeulenrode, Germany) and the AirHeel (Aircast/Donjoy, Vista, California) (see Box 2). However, no rigorous controlled studies have validated their use.

Aprotinin

Aprotinin is a naturally occurring broad-spectrum protease derived from bovine lung. It has been hypothesized that it may be used to treat tendinopathies by its action of inhibiting the inflammatory proteases that degrade tendons. Initial results seemed promising with 78% of patients returning promptly to sporting activities following a course of injections as compared with 30% in the placebo group [69]. However, in a prospective, randomized, double-blind study by Brown and colleagues [70], there was no statistically significant improvement in symptomatology and function, although there was a trend toward significant improvement in the Victorian Institute of Sports Assessment—Achilles (VISA-A) score at 12 months in the treatment group. In a review of 422 injections, Orchard and colleagues [71] found a systemic allergy rate of 2.6% upon reexposure.

Physical therapy modalities

Therapeutic ultrasound. Therapeutic ultrasound has been shown in vitro to promote earlier resolution of inflammation, an increased rate of angiogenesis, denser collagen fibers, and increased tissue strength [72]. Over 1 million treatments per year involve its use [73]. However, in two meta-analyses [74,75], no robust evidence was found to support its use. In spite of the theoretical benefits of therapeutic ultrasound, better in vivo evidence is necessary before its use can be recommended.

Extracorporeal shock wave therapy. Extracorporeal shock wave therapy (ESWT) is a modality most commonly used within orthopaedics in the treatment of fracture nonunion and calcific tendonitis. Proponents of its use suggest that it has a role in the treatment of soft tissue pathologies, including tendinopathies. However, the mechanism of action is unknown, with hypotheses involving increased diffusion of cytokines across vessel walls as a consequence of the energy delivered, resulting in the stimulation of angiogenesis and healing [76]. A recent randomized placebo-controlled trial showed no difference in pain relief and could not recommend its use in the treatment of chronic Achilles tendon pain [77]. The only robust study showing benefits of ESWT was by Rompe and colleagues [78], who found no difference in VISA-A and Likert scoring at 4 months' follow-up between those treated by ESWT and those treated by eccentric loading physical therapy. However, they also found that ESWT and physical therapy were significantly better than a wait-and-see policy. Further research with larger sample sizes is therefore necessary to clarify any potential benefits of this treatment.

Low-level laser therapy. Low-level laser therapy is another physical treatment applied to soft tissue disorders. One study involving seven patients demonstrated a decrease in intratendinous concentrations of prostaglandin E2 as compared with a placebo group treated with sham laser [79]. However, studies have generally been of small size and contradictory in their findings. The use of low-level laser therapy cannot be advocated until more evidence is presented [80].

Cryotherapy. The use of cryotherapy in acute sports injuries is widespread and certainly has analgesic properties [81,82]. There is some pathological evidence of decreased capillary blood flow, preserved deep oxygen tension, and facilitated venous capillary outflow. In spite of this relatively sound pathological basis, there is no clinical evidence for its ongoing use in Achilles tendinopathy.

Manual and physical therapies

Variations in deep transverse friction massage therapy, such as the Cyriax method, have gained more recent popularity, especially amongst physical therapists. Some animal models have shown some pathological basis for their use [83,84]. However, a Cochrane review of their use in all tendinopathies did not show any consistent benefit, although these failings may be in at least part due to the small sample sizes in these series [85]. However, one more recent study did show a decrease in stretch reflex amplitude as well as some improvement in stiffness and pain with a variation of this method [86].

Physical therapy training programs have been a mainstay in the treatment of Achilles tendinopathy. The importance of eccentric training was first stressed in the early 1980s [87]. The pilot study by Alfredson and colleagues [88] showed that at 12 weeks all 15 patients had returned to preinjury-level activity status (although 1 patient later relapsed and required surgery). All these patients had been previously treated with the usual gamut of nonoperative therapies—rest, NSAIDS, change of shoes, orthoses—without success and were on the waiting list for surgery. Following treatment, the mean visual analog scale (VAS) score decreased from 81.2 to 4.8 in this cohort. A larger study showed satisfactory results in 90 out of 101 tendons, although rates were far lower (32%) when this method was used for treatment of insertional Achilles tendonitis [89,90]. A further multicenter randomized prospective study was undertaken to compare the results of eccentric and concentric training regimes. The study showed that 81% of the eccentric training group were satisfied and had returned to previous activity levels compared with only 38% in the concentric training group. This evidence was further reinforced by an ultrasonographical study with 3.8 years' follow-up [91]. This found that the hypoechoic areas and irregular structure had resolved in 19 out of 26 patients using an eccentric training program. Rompe and colleagues [78] demonstrated that eccentric training had significantly better results in outcome measures (VISA-A and Linker scale) as compared with a wait-and-see policy. In a study of eccentric training in nonathletic patients, however, Sayana and colleagues [92] found a less optimistic outcome with the exercise program only being effective in 56% of patients. It has also been the authors' experience that more sedentary patients have more difficulty in completing eccentric training programs with results that, while favorable, are not as good as those in athletic patients.

Alfredson's regime. A patient following Alfredson's regime performs three sets of 15 eccentric heel drops. This exercise is usually performed on a stair with the patient standing on the ventral halves of his or her feet, the uninjured foot on an upper stair and the injured foot on a lower stair [93]. The patient starts by lifting his body with the uninjured foot so that the injured ankle is plantarflexed. Then the heel of the injured foot is lowered below the level of the stair and the front of the foot, thus loading the calf eccentrically. The exercise can be done with the knee either flexed, to load the soleus components, or extended, to load the gastrocnemius components. These sets are performed twice daily, 7 days a week for 12 weeks (Figs. 3 and 4).

The exercise is intended to be painful. When the exercise can be performed without pain, extra load is given to reach "a new level of painful training."

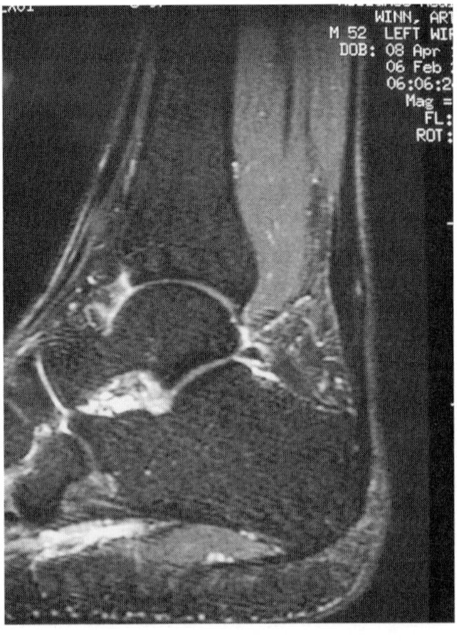

Fig. 3. MRI T2-weighted image showing typical appearances of tendinopathy with high signal seen within the tendon.

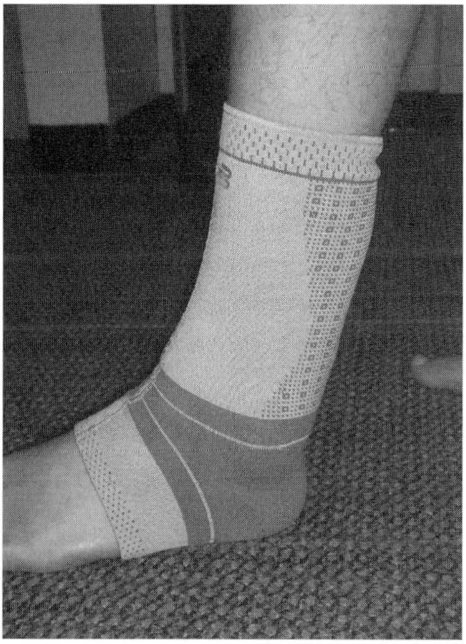

Fig. 4. Patient wearing Achillotrain brace-Bauerfiend.

There is no convincing theory of why this method should work. Doppler and ultrasound studies have shown reduced neovascularization in the treated patients and postulated that these "neovessels" and accompanying nerves were the source of the pain [94]. To test this hypothesis, a sclerosing agent (polidocanol) was injected ventral to the tendon in the area of neovascularization. The early results appear promising with 8 out of 10 patients symptom-free at 2 years following two injections with an ultrasonically confirmed return to normality in tendon morphology. A larger randomized study is to follow [95]. This theory and findings would therefore contradict most widely held opinion and treatments that aim to stimulate angiogenesis in the area of tendinopathy that corresponds to a zone of relative hypovascularity—thus the paradox of Achilles tendinopathy.

Operative treatments

While there have been no prospective randomized controlled studies comparing different operative treatments or operative with conservative treatments, surgery is still considered a reasonable alternative after a failed nonoperative regime. Likewise, various techniques and approaches have been described. Again, the mechanism whereby surgical interventions work remain unclear.

It has also, reasonably, been postulated that the success following surgery may in the most part be due to the enforced postoperative rest and relative immobilization, followed by controlled rehabilitation.

Open surgery

Open adhesiolysis, plus tendon debridement if required, is the most commonly used surgical technique for treatment of Achilles tendinopathy (Figs. 5 and 6). This technique employs a longitudinal approach, which may be midline, medial, or lateral [65,96], depending upon the intended procedure and preoperative investigations. Simple division of adhesions of the paratenon or debridement of the paratenon would lend itself to a midline approach: The crural fascia is incised and any adhesions in the paratenon and the crural fascia are carefully excised. If there is any central core degeneration upon preoperative imaging, the paratenon and the tendon are incised, the affected portion is then resected, and the defect in the tendon repaired by simple side-to-side suturing. If this degeneration is not present on imaging, then, theoretically, longitudinal tenotomies may be beneficial in promoting neoangiogenesis and tendon healing [8,97].

If a preoperative MRI shows that resection of large areas of degeneration is necessary and augmentation will be required, then a medial or lateral approach would depend upon whether the surgeon prefers to harvest flexor halluicis longus (FHL) or peroneus brevis. Also, if during debridement of core degeneration more than 50% of the tendon is excised, then augmentation may be necessary [98]. FHL is most commonly used for augmentation, although some advocate the use of peroneus brevis [8]. FHL may be locally harvested in the posterior compartment of the lower leg and fixed to the

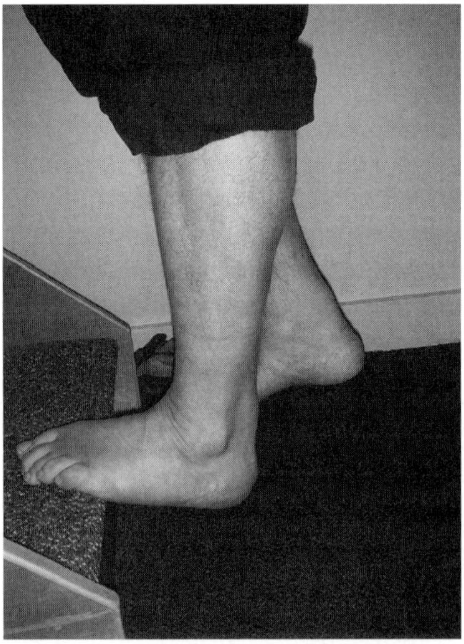

Fig. 5. Alfredson's regime: knee extended.

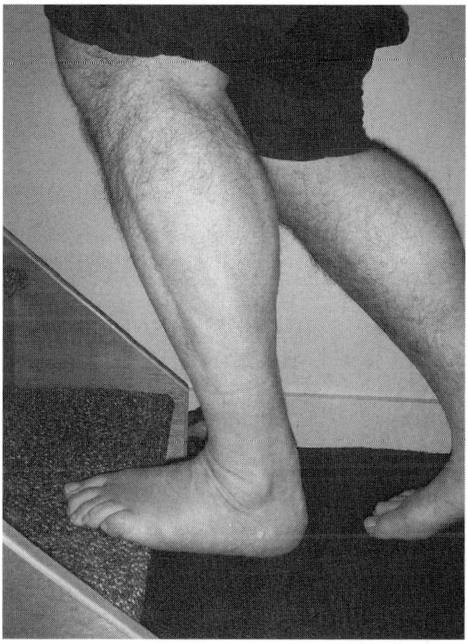

Fig. 6. Alfredson's regime: knee flexed.

calcaneus by a variety of methods. Another option is to make a second incision in the midfoot to harvest greater length so that FHL may be passed through a drill-hole in the calcaneus and looped up to attach to the lateral side of the Achilles tendon. This can, however, make the repair quite bulky. There is no published data on whether this provides any clinical or mechanical benefit. It has been hypothesized that the use of FHL is not without morbidity in the elite athlete [8], although the authors are not aware of any substantive data to support this.

Achilles-tendon–bone allografts have been used for the treatment of significant tendon defects, usually in cases of neglected Achilles tendon ruptures [99–101]. This technique may also be used in the severe recalcitrant tendinopathy where the structure of the entire distal tendon has been compromised. The Achilles tendon is resected up to the required level and a trough is created in the host calcaneus to receive the allograft bone. The graft is attached distally (bone to bone) by two 4.0-mm screws. Proximally it is attached (tendon to tendon) by interrupted nonabsorbable sutures under sufficient tension as to place the foot in a position that is slightly more equinus than that of the unaffected foot. Although only a few cases have been performed, results have been encouraging in what are very challenging cases. The associated pain relief probably relates to the debridement of the associated nocioceptors in the diseased tissue.

Overall surgical intervention is deemed to have a success rate of 43% to 100% [7,13,24,41–53]. However a review of 26 studies reporting surgical outcomes by Tallon and colleagues [102] found that the methodology scores of these studies as a whole was low with a negative correlation between reported success rate and overall method scores. However, they do acknowledge that study methods have improved over the past 20 years. A more recent prospective study by Paavola and colleagues [42] found that 94% of patients operated on for Achilles tendinopathy without an intratendinous lesion (group A) had mild or no symptoms. In those with an intratendinous lesion (group B) the rate was 79%. Patients in group A had a higher chance of recovery of sporting activity (88% versus 54%).

Postoperative rehabilitation. There is as much variation and poor information about postoperative rehabilitation as about the other facets of noninsertional Achilles tendinopathy.

Immobilization in a cast or boot is recommended from 2 to 8 weeks and the degree of weight-bearing allowed is also variable. However, the exact protocol is bound to vary and be very much dependent upon the procedure performed. For example, protocols could vary according to the amount of tendon resected and whether or not wound problems are anticipated. What is known, however, is that controlled stretching on collagen synthesis during the inflammatory phase of healing has beneficial effects that result in improved fiber alignment and increases tensile strength [36]. Also, collagen that remains unstressed in the proliferative and remodelling phases is haphazard in organization and tends to be weaker in terms of tensile strength. Thus, early mobilization regimes are beneficial following tendon repair and tenocyte function even though the exact mechanism of action in unknown [103].

In the uncomplicated case with no anticipated wound problems and minimal tendon resection, the authors use the following regime:

- Two weeks in protective cast (either plaster of Paris back, U slabs, or lightweight cast) and protected weight-bearing (ie, crutches with the foot in the midrange of plantarflexion).
- Review of wound at 2 weeks. If satisfactory, then supervised rehabilitation commences with physiotherapists. The amount of protection required at this stage depends upon the exact procedure undertaken and is thus "individualized."
- Repairs requiring tendon augments are immobilized in a range-of-motion walker with a block to dorsiflexion for a further 4 weeks while active plantarflexion exercises are commenced, again with protected weight-bearing.
- Following a simple adhesiolysis and minimum tendon debridement, weight-bearing occurs as tolerated once the wound has healed and rehabilitation also occurs at a pace tolerable to the patient with early commencement of eccentric exercises.

Percutaneous tenotomies

Percutaneous tenotomies, with or without ultrasound guidance, may be used in the treatment of isolated well-defined nodular Achilles tendinopathy [24,103]. For best results, a percutaneous tenotomy should be performed in the absence of concomitant paratendinopathy. It is possible to perform percutaneous tenotomy in the outpatient setting under local anesthetic without a tourniquet [8]. A rating of good or excellent in 75% of patients at a mean of 51 months' follow-up has been reported. However 56% of those rated as good or fair underwent formal open exploration of the Achilles tendon within a year. The investigators report this to be a successful technique that involves minimal complications and does not hinder any required further surgery. However, 11% of patients were rated as having a poor outcome and the authors believe that this should be discussed as part of the consent process.

Tenoscopy

Arthroscopic treatment of conditions around the hindfoot is becoming more widespread and the attraction of a successful minimally invasive treatment is obvious. Steenstra and van Dijk [53] reported the results of Achilles tenoscopy in a cohort of 20 patients at a mean of 6 years' follow-up. Epidural, spinal, or general anesthetic and a tourniquet are necessary for this day-case surgical technique. A 2.7-mm 30° oblique or a standard 4-mm arthroscope is used with irrigation (gravity maintained or under pressure). The aim of this procedure is to remove all areas of inflamed paratenon and neovascularization as well as to free up the plantaris tendon. A full radius 2.7-mm resector shaver is used through a distal (2–3 cm distal to the pathological thickened nodule) and proximal (2–4 cm cranial) portal. All patients had significant relief with most being able to resume sporting activities (as early as 4–8 weeks). There were no complications. Although the results are certainly encouraging, further prospective randomized evidence is necessary together with larger sample sizes.

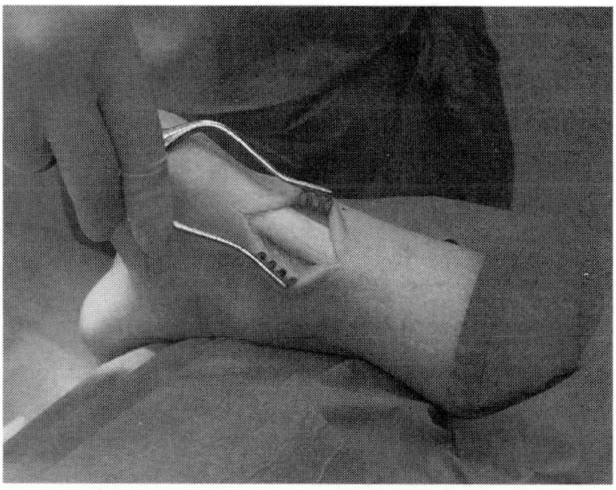

Fig. 7. Typical appearance at surgery during open adhesiolysis, the most commonly used surgical technique for treatment of Achilles tendinopathy.

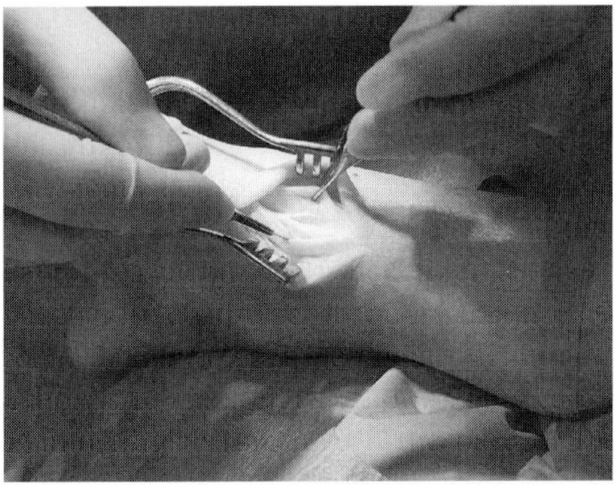

Fig. 8. Typical appearance at surgery.

Results

Paavola and colleagues [51] reported a complication rate of 11% in a study of 432 surgically treated cases. These included (in descending order of frequency) skin edge necrosis, superficial wound infection, seroma or hematoma formation, sural neuritis, new partial rupture, and thrombosis. Overall wound problems constituted 56% of complications. A further study by Paavola and colleagues [42] showed a complication rate of 6% if paratendinous adhesionolysis was performed, but this rose to 27% if excision of a segment of core degeneration was undertaken.

In a long-term study with a mean follow-up of 5 years, 92% of patients were satisfied and had returned to their desired level of activity post–surgical-treatment [104]. However, they also discovered that peak eccentric and concentric torque was significantly lower (7.2%–8.8%) on the treated side as compared with the other leg, although this difference was asymptomatic. Most of the literature supports a surgical success rate of 75% to 100%. However Maffulli and colleagues [49] showed that this success rate depends upon the chronicity of symptoms. Their 35-month follow-up of 14 athletes with an average of 87 months of symptoms showed a success rate of 43% with central core decompression. This would appear to support the practice of more prompt surgical referral in the event of failure of conservative treatment.

Summary

Noninsertional Achilles tendinopathy is an increasingly common condition. It is a degenerative rather than an inflammatory condition and is usually related to overuse. The mainstay of treatment remains nonoperative, involving correction of any precipitating factors if at all possible. Eccentric exercise programs and more directed rehabilitation are giving good to excellent results. Surgical treatment also appears to produce good results but the authors are uncertain of exactly how or why.

Neither different operative techniques nor nonoperative regimes have been subjected to controlled trials. Rather, the condition is still treated on the basis of anecdotal evidence combined with personal experience. However, increased knowledge of the basic science of tendinopathy and tendon healing has directed therapeutic regimens and will continue to do so. Manipulation of proteolytic enzymes and control of neovascularization are probably the two areas that show most promise (Figs. 7 and 8).

References

[1] Homer. The Iliad. Nagles R, (trans). New York: Viking; 1996.
[2] Paavola M, Jarvinen TAH. Paratendinopathy. Foot Ankle Clin 2005;2:279–92.
[3] Maffulli N, Khan KM, Puddu G. Overuse tendon conditions: time to change a confusing terminology. Arthroscopy 1998;14:840–3.
[4] Leadbetter W. Soft tissue athletic injury in sports injuries: mechanisms, prevention and treatment. Baltimore (MD): Williams & Wilkins; 1994.
[5] Sports-induced inflammation. Clinical and basic science concepts (symposium series). Park Ridge (IL): American Academy of Orthopaedic Surgeons; 1990.
[6] Alfredson H, Thorsen K, Lorentzon R. In situ microdialysis in tendon tissue: high levels of glutamate, but not prostaglandin E2 in chronic Achilles tendon pain. Knee Surg Sports Traumatol Arthrosc 1999;7:378–81.
[7] Maffulli N, Kader D. Tendinopathy of the tendo achillis. J Bone Joint Surg Br 2002;84:1–8.
[8] Vora AM, Myerson MS, Maffulli N. Tendinopathy of the main body of the Achilles tendon. Foot Ankle Clin 2005;10:293–308.
[9] Johansson C. Injuries in elite orienteers. Am J Sports Med 1986;14:410–5.
[10] Lysholm J, Wiklander J. Injuries in runners. Am J Sports Med 1987;15:168–71.
[11] Murray IR, Murray SA, MacKenzie K, et al. How evidence based is the management of two common sports injuries in a sports injury clinic? Br J Sports Med 2005;39:912–6.
[12] James SL, Bates BT, Osterling LR. Injuries to runners. Am J Sports Med 1978;6:40–50.
[13] Kvist M. Achilles tendon injuries in athletes. Sports Med 1994;18:173–201.
[14] el Hawary R, Stanish WD, Curwin SL. Rehabilitation of tendon injuries in sport. Sports Med 1997;24:347–58.
[15] Barfred T. Experimental rupture of Achilles tendon. Acta Orthop Scand 1971;42:528–43.
[16] Benjamin M, Evans EJ, Copp L. The histology of tendon attachment to bone in man. J Anat 1986;149:89–100.
[17] Schepsis AA. Achilles tendon disorders in athletes. Am J Sports Med 2002;30(2):287–305.
[18] Carr AJ, Norris SH. The blood supply of the calcaneal tendon. J Bone Joint Surg Br 1989; 71:100–1.
[19] Lagergren C, Lindholm A. Vascular distribution in the Achilles tendon. An angiographic and microangiographic study. Acta Chir Scand 1958;116:491–6.
[20] Astrom M, Westlin N. Blood flow in the human Achilles tendon assessed by laser flowmetry. J Orthop Res 1994;12:246–52.
[21] Kannus P, Jozsa L, Jarvinnen M. Basic science of tendons. In: Garrett WE Jr, Speer KP, Kirkendall DT, editors. Principles and practice of orthopaedic sports medicine. Philadelphia: Lippincott Williams and Wilkins; 2000. p. 21–37.
[22] Williams SK, Brage M. Heel pain—plantar fasciitis and Achilles enthesopathy. Clin Sports Med 2004;23:123–44.
[23] Soma CA, Mandelbaum BR. Achilles tendon disorders. Clin Sports Med 1994;13:811–23.

[24] Clement DB, Taunton J, Smart GW. A survey of overuse running injuries. Physician Sportsmed 1981;9:47–58.
[25] Smart GW, Taunton JE, Clement DB. Achilles tendon disorders in runners: a review. Med Sci Sports Exerc 1980;12:231–43.
[26] Hart DA, Frank CB, Bray RC. Inflammatory processes in repetitive motion and overuse syndromes; potential role of neurogenic mechanisms in tendons and ligaments. In: Gordon SL, Blair SJ, Fine LJ, editors. Repetitive motion disorders of the upper extremity. Rosemont (IL): Am Academy Orthop Surgeons; 1995. p. 247–62.
[27] Khan KM, Cook JL, Bonar F, et al. Histopathology of common tendinopathies. Update and implications for clinical management. Sports Med 1999;27:393–408.
[28] Kannus P. Etiology and pathophysiology of chronic tendon disorders in sports. Scand J Med Sci Sports 1997;7:78–85.
[29] Jarvinen TAH, Kannus P, Jozsa I, et al. Achilles tendon injuries. Curr Opin Rheumatol 2001;13:150–5.
[30] Magra M, Maffulli N. Molecular events in tendinopathy: a role for metalloproteases. Foot Ankle Clin 2005;10:267–77.
[31] Langberg H, Bulow J, Kjaer M. Blood in the peritendinous space of the human Achilles tendon during exercise. Acta Physiol Scand 1998;163:149–53.
[32] Ahmed IM, Lagopoulos M, McConnell P, et al. Blood supply of the Achilles tendon. J Orthop Res 1998;16(5):591–6.
[33] Kvist M, Jozsa L, Jarvinen M. Vascular changes in the ruptured Achilles tendon and paratenon. Int Orthop 1992;16(4):377–82.
[34] Zantop T, Tillmann B, Petersen W. Quantitative assessment of blood vessels of the human Achilles tendon: an immunohistochemical cadaver study. Arch Orthop Trauma Surg 2003; 123(9):501–4.
[35] McGarvey WC, Singh D, Trevino S. Partial Achilles tendon ruptures associated with fluoroquinolone antibiotics: a case report and literature review. Foot Ankle Int 1996;8:496–8.
[36] Parmar C, Hennessy MS. Achilles tendon rupture following combination therapy with steroids and levofloxacin: case series and review of the literature. Foot Ankle Int, in press.
[37] Bestwick CS, Maffulli N. Reactive oxygen species and tendon problems: review and hypothesis. Sports Med Arthroscopy Rev 2000;8:6–16.
[38] Lin J, Fessell DP, Jacobsen JA, et al. An illustrated tutorial of musculoskeletal sonosgraphy part 1, introduction and general principle. AJR Am J Roentgenol 2000;175:637–45.
[39] Khan KM, Forster BB, Robinson J, et al. Are ultrasound and magnetic resonance imaging of value in assessment of Achilles tendon disorders? A two year prospective study. Br J Sports Med 2003;37:149–53.
[40] Paavola M, Kannus P, Paakkala T, et al. Long term prognosis of patients with Achilles tendinopathy. An observational 8-year follow-up study. Am J Sports Med 2000;28:634–42.
[41] Leppilahti J, Karpakka J, Gorra A, et al. Surgical treatment of overuse injuries to the Achilles tendon. Clin J Sport Med 1994;4:100–7.
[42] Paavola M, Kannus P, Orava S, et al. surgical treatment for chronic Achilles tendinopathy: a prospective 7 month follow-up study. Br J Sports Med 2002;36:178–82.
[43] Rolf C, Movin T. Etiology, histology and outcome of surgery in achillodynia. Foot Ankle Int 1997;18:565–9.
[44] Johnston E, Scranton P Jr, Pfeffer GB. Chronic disorders of the Achilles tendon: results of conservative and surgical treatments. Foot Ankle Int 1997;18:570–4.
[45] Astrom M. Partial rupture in chronic Achilles tendinopathy. A retrospective analysis of 342 cases. Acta Orthop Scand 1998;69(4):404–7.
[46] Binfield PM, Malluffi N. Surgical treatment of common tendinopathies of the lower limb. Sports Exerc Injury 1997;3:116–22.
[47] Lehto MU, Jarvinen M, Suominen P. Chronic Achilles peritendinitis and retrocalcanear bursitis. Long term follow-up of surgically treated cases. Knee Surg Sports Traumatol Arthrosc 1994;2:182–5.

[48] Saltzman CL, Tearse DS. Achilles tendon injuries. J Am Acad Orthop Surg 1998;6:316–25.
[49] Maffulli N, Binfield PM, Moore D, et al. Surgical decompression of chronic central core lesions of the Achilles tendon. Am J Sports Med 1999;27(6):747–52.
[50] Morberg P, Jerre R, Sward L, et al. Long-term results after surgical management of partial Achilles tendon ruptures. Scand J Med Sci Sports 1997;7:299–303.
[51] Paavola M, Orava S, Leppilahti J, et al. Chronic Achilles tendon overuse injury: complications after surgical treatment. Am J Sports Med 2000;28:77–82.
[52] Sandmeier R, Renstrom PA. Diagnosis and treatment of chronic tendon disorders in sports. Scand J Med Sci Sports 1997;7:96–106.
[53] Steenstra F, van Dijk N. Achilles tenoscopy. Foot Ankle Clin N Am 2006;11:429–38.
[54] Rees JD, Wilson AM, Wolman RL. Current concepts in the management of tendon disorders. Rheumatology 2006;45:508–21.
[55] Tsai WC, Hsu CC, Chou SW, et al. Effects of celecoxib on migration, proliferation and collagen expression of tendon cells. Connect Tissue Res 2007;48(1):46–51.
[56] Forslund C, Bylander B, Aspenburg P. Indomethacin and celecoxib improve tendon healing in rats. Acta Orthop Scand 2003;74(4):465–9.
[57] Thomas J, Taylor D, Crowell R, et al. The effect of indomethacin on Achilles tendon healing in rabbits. Clin Orthop Relat Res 1991;272:308–11.
[58] Marsolais D, Cote CH, Frenette J. Nonsteroidal anti-inflammatory drug reduces neutrophil and macrophage accumulation but does not improve tendon regeneration. Lab Invest 2003;83(7):991–9.
[59] Alfredson H. Chronic midportion Achilles tendinopathy: an update on research and treatment. Clin Sports Med 2003;4:727–41.
[60] Weiler JM. Medical modifiers of sports injury. The use of nonsteroidal anti-inflammatory drugs (NSAIDs) in sports soft tissue injury. Clin Sports Med 1992;11:625–44.
[61] McLaughlin GJ, Handoll HHG. Interventions for treating acute and chronic Achilles tendonitis. The Cochrane Database Syst Rev 2007;2:CD000232.
[62] Galloway MT, Jokl P, Dayton OW. Achilles tendon overuse injuries. Clin Sports Med 1992;11(4):771–82.
[63] Ljungqvist R. Subcutaneous partial rupture of the Achilles tendon. Acta Orthop Scand Suppl 1968;113:1–86.
[64] Williams JGP. Achilles tendon lesions in sport. Sports Med 1986;3:114–35.
[65] Shrier I, Matheson GO, Kohl HW 3rd. Achilles tendonitis: Are corticosteroid injections useful or harmful? Clin J Sport Med 1996;6(4):245–50.
[66] Gill SS, Gelbke MK, Mattson SL, et al. Fluoroscopically guided low-volume peritendinous corticosteroid injection for Achilles tendinopathy. A safety study. J Bone Joint Surg Am 2004;86(4):802–6.
[67] Paoloni JA, Appleyard RC, Nelson J, et al. Topical glceryl trinitrate treatment of chronic noninsertional Achilles tendinopathy. J Bone Joint Surg Am 2004;86:916–22.
[68] Lowdon A, Bader DL, Mowat AG. The effect of heel pads on the treatment of Achilles tendonitis: a double blind trial. Am J Sports Med 1984;12(6):431–5.
[69] Capasso G, Maffulli N, Testa V, et al. Preliminary results with peritendinous protease inhibitor infections in the treatment of Achilles tendonitis. J Sports Traumatol Rel Res 1993; 15:37–43.
[70] Brown R, Orchard J, Kinchington M, et al. Aprotinin in the management of Achilles tendinopathy: a randomised control trial. Br J Sports Med 2006;40(3):275–9.
[71] Orchard J, Hofman J, Brown R. The risks of local aprotinin injections for the treatment of chronic tendinopathy. Sports Health 2005;23:24–8.
[72] Speed CA. Therapeutic ultrasound in soft tissue lesions. Rheumatology 2001;40:1331–6.
[73] ter Haar G, Dyson M, Oakley EM. The use of ultrasound by physiotherapists in Britain. Ultrasound Med Biol 1985;13:659–63.
[74] Beckerman H, Bouter LM, van der Heijdan, et al. Efficacy of physiotherapy for musculoskeletal disorders: What can we learn from research? Br J Gen Pract 1993;43:73–7.

[75] Gam AN, Johannsen F. Ultrasound therapy in musculoskeletal disorders: a meta-analysis. Pain 1995;63:85–91.
[76] Sems A, Dimeff R, Ianotti JP. Extracorporeal shock wave therapy in the treatment of chronic tendinopathies. J Am Acad Orthop Surg 2006;14:195–204.
[77] Costa ML, Shepstone L, Donell ST, et al. Shock wave therapy for chronic Achilles tendon pain: a randomized placebo-controlled trial. Clin Orthop Relat Res 2005;440:199–204.
[78] Rompe JD, Nafe B, Furia JP, et al. Eccentric loading, shock-wave treatment, or a wait-and-see policy for tendinopathy of the main body of tendo Achillis: a randomised controlled trial. Am J Sports Med 2007;35(3):374–83.
[79] Bjordal JM, Lopes-Martins RAB, Iverson VV. A randomised, placebo controlled trial of low level laser therapy for activated Achilles tendonitis with microdialysis measurement of peritendinous prostoglandin E2 concentrations. Br J Sports Med 2006;40:76–80.
[80] Basford JR. Low intensity laser therapy: still not an established clinical tool. Lasers Surg Med 1995;16:331–42.
[81] Knobloch K, Graseman R, Jagodzinski M, et al. Changes of Achilles midportion microcirculation after repetitive simultaneous cryotherapy and compression after using a Cryo/Cuff. Am J Sports Med 2006;34(12):1953–9.
[82] Knobloch K, Grasemann R, Spies M, et al. Intermittent Koldblue (R) cryotherapy of 3 × 10 min changes mid-portion Achilles tendon microcirculation. Br J Sports Med 2007;41:e4.
[83] Davidson CJ, Ganion LR, Gehlsen GM, et al. Rat tendon morphologic and functional changes resulting from soft tissue mobilization. Med Sci Sports Exerc 1997;29:313–9.
[84] Gehlsen GM, Ganion LR, Helfst R. Fibroblast responses to variation in soft tissue mobilization pressure. Med Sci Sports Exerc 1999;31:531–5.
[85] Brousseau L, Casimiro L, Milne S, et al. Deep transverse friction massage for treating tendonitis. Cochrane Database Syst Rev 2002;4:CD003528.
[86] Howell JN, Cabell KS, Chila AG, et al. Stretch reflex and Hoffmann reflex responses to osteopathic manipulative treatment in subjects with Achilles tendinitis. J Am Osteopath Assoc 2006;106(9):537–45.
[87] Curvin S, Stanish WD. Tendinitis: its etiology and treatment. Lexington (KY): Collamore Press, DC Heath & Co.; 1984.
[88] Alfredson H, Pietila T, Johnsson P, et al. Heavy-load eccentric calf muscle training for the treatment of chronic Achilles tendinosis. Am J Sports Med 1998;26(3):360–6.
[89] Fahlstrom M, Jonsson P, Lorentzon R, et al. Chronic Achilles tendon pain treated with eccentric calf-muscle training. Knee Surg Sports Traumatol Arthrosc 2001;9:42–7.
[90] Mafi N, Lorentzon R, Alfredson H. Superior results with eccentric calf-muscle training compared to concentric training in a randomized prospective multi-center study on patients with chronic Achilles tendinosis. Knee Surg Sports Traumatol Arthrosc 2003;11: 327–33.
[91] Ohberg L, Lorentzon R, Alfredson H. Eccentric training in patients with chronic Achilles tendinosis: normalized tendon structure and decreased thickness at follow up. Br J Sports Med 2004;38:8–11.
[92] Sayana MK, Maffulli N. Eccentric calf muscle training in non-athletic patients with Achilles tendinopathy. J Sci Med Sport 2007;10(1):52–8.
[93] Alfredson H. Conservative Management of Achilles tendinopathy: new ideas. Foot Ankle Clin 2005;10:321–9.
[94] Ohberg L, Alfredson H. Effects on neovascularisation behind the good results with eccentric training in chronic mid-portion Achilles tendinosis? Knee Surg Sports Traumatol Arthrosc 2001;12:465–70.
[95] Ohberg L, Alfredson H. Ultrasound guided sclerosing of neovessels in painful chronic Achilles tendinosis: pilot study of a new treatment. Br J Sports Med 2002;36:173–7.
[96] Schepsis AA, Leach RE. Surgical management of Achilles tendonitis. Am J Sports Med 1987;15:308–15.

[97] Friedrich T, Schmidt W, Jungmichel D, et al. Histopathology in rabbit Achilles tendon after operative tenolysis (longitudinal fiber incisions). Scand J Med Sci Sports 2001;11:4–8.
[98] Den Hartog BD. Flexor hallucis longus transfer for chronic Achilles tendonosis. Foot Ankle Int 2003;24(3):233–7.
[99] Haraguchi N, Bluman EM, Myerson MS. Reconstruction of chronic Achilles tendon disorders with Achilles tendon allograft. Techniques Foot Ankle Surg 2005;4(3):154–9.
[100] Nellas ZJ, Loder BG, Wertheimer SJ. Reconstruction of an Achilles tendon defect utilizing an Achilles tendon allograft. J Foot Ankle Surg 1996;35:144–8.
[101] Yuen JC, Nicholas R. Reconstruction of a total Achilles tendon and soft-tissue defect using an Achilles allograft combined with a rectus muscle free flap. Plast Reconstr Surg 2001;107:1807–11.
[102] Tallon C, Coleman BD, Khan KM, et al. Outcome of surgery for chronic Achilles tendinopathy. A critical review. Am J Sports Med 2001;29:315–20.
[103] Buckwalter JA. Effects of early motion on healing of musculoskeletal tissues. Hand Clin 1996;12:13–24.
[104] Ohberg L, Lorentzon R, Alfredson H. Good clinical results but persisting side-to-side differences in calf muscle strength after surgical treatment of chronic Achilles tendinosis-a 5 year follow up. Scand J Med Sci Sports 2001;11(4):207–12.

ELSEVIER
SAUNDERS

Foot Ankle Clin N Am
12 (2007) 643–657

FOOT AND
ANKLE CLINICS

Acute and Chronic Peroneal Tendon Dislocations

Peter Rosenfeld, MB, BS, FRCS (Tr&Orth)

St Mary's Hospital, Paddington, London W2 1NY, England

Peroneal tendon dislocation is easily misdiagnosed as an ankle sprain and, as such, is often mistreated. Most such injuries are due to sports trauma, particularly skiing, and occur in forced dorsiflexion of the ankle joint. Because the ankle is tender laterally with swelling and lateral ecchymosis, the injury is often misinterpreted as an anterior talofibular ligament injury. Untreated, peroneal tendon dislocation frequently becomes a chronic dislocation, causing significant pain and activity limitation. Peroneal tendon dislocation is an uncommon injury and was first reported by Monteggia in 1803 [1], occurring in a ballet dancer. It is more commonly associated with a wide variety of sports, including skiing, soccer, basketball, rugby, cycling, rowing, baseball, and horse riding [2–8]. Over 92% of cases are secondary to trauma [9] with the remaining congenital cases thought to be due to a deficiency in the bony or soft tissue restraints [10]. Acute peroneal dislocation is very common in calcaneal fractures and occurs in up to 40% of intra-articular fractures [11]. Clinical diagnosis of the acute injury can be difficult or uncertain and is reliably confirmed on MRI or volume-rendered CT images. Operative repair of the acute injury is generally recommended because conservative measures have a high recurrence rate [12]. The surgical procedures can be divided into five main categories: (1) superior peroneal retinaculum (SPR) reattachment, (2) SPR reconstruction, (3) rerouting procedures, (4) bone block procedures, and (5) groove-deepening procedures. Postoperative immobilization for 6 weeks is recommended and the results of surgery have a high success rate with some minor complications [2–8, 12–24].

E-mail address: pfrosenfeld@btinternet.com

doi:10.1016/j.fcl.2007.07.001

Anatomy

The peroneal tendons (longus and brevis) lie within a fibro-osseous tunnel as they course behind and under the distal fibula. The tunnel, formed by the fibula, the tendon sheath, and the SPR, is supported inferiorly by the calcaneofibular ligament (CFL) (Fig. 1).

The SPR, a condensation of layers from the superficial fascia of the leg and the peroneal tendon sheath, starts 2 cm above the tip of the fibula. The SPR originates from the periosteum of the fibula, is 1 to 2 cm wide, and forms two bands, one running posteriorly into the Achilles tendon sheath and the other running inferiorly to insert into the calcaneum. The inferior peroneal retinaculum starts 2 cm distal to the tip of the fibula and continues into the inferior extensor retinaculum.

The fibula groove is formed by the bony contour of the fibula and the overlying specialized periosteum proximally. Distally the fibula is convex with the groove formed by specialized periosteum, which forms a thick fibrocartilagenous groove. The fibrocartilage has a prominent lateral ridge, which deepens the groove by 1 to 2 mm. The SPR attaches to this lateral ridge. A smaller medial ridge receives the posterior talofibular ligament and the posterior syndesmotic ligaments [25] (Fig. 2).

The bony contour of the posterior fibula can be variable, as noted by Edwards [26] in a study of 178 cadaveric fibulae, with 82% having a shallow posterior groove, 11% having a flat posterior surface (no groove), and 7% having a convex surface throughout.

Mechanism

Most cases are secondary to ankle trauma, with congenital or atraumatic examples much less frequent [7,22]. Dislocation of the tendons is most often

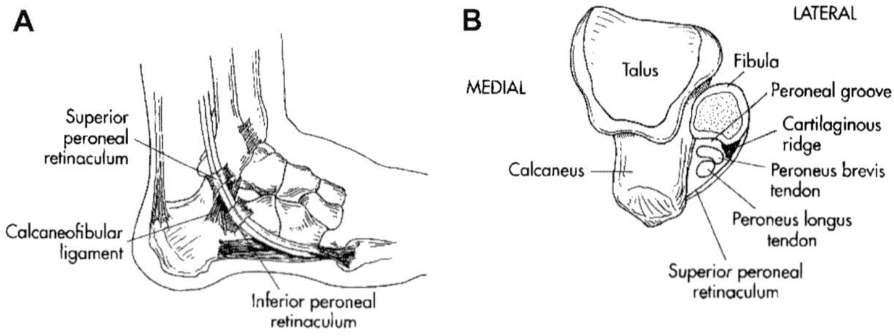

Fig. 1. Anatomic relationship of ankle with peroneal tendons held in position by superior and inferior peroneal retinacula and by fibrous rim on posterolateral aspect of fibula. Calcaneofibula ligament lies below peroneal tendons. (*A*) Lateral view. (*B*) Superior view. (*From* Clanton TO. Athletic injuries to the soft tissues of the foot and ankle. In: Coughlin MJ, Mann RA, editors. Surgery of the foot and ankle. 7th edition. St. Louis (MO): Mosby; 1999. p. 1158; with permission.)

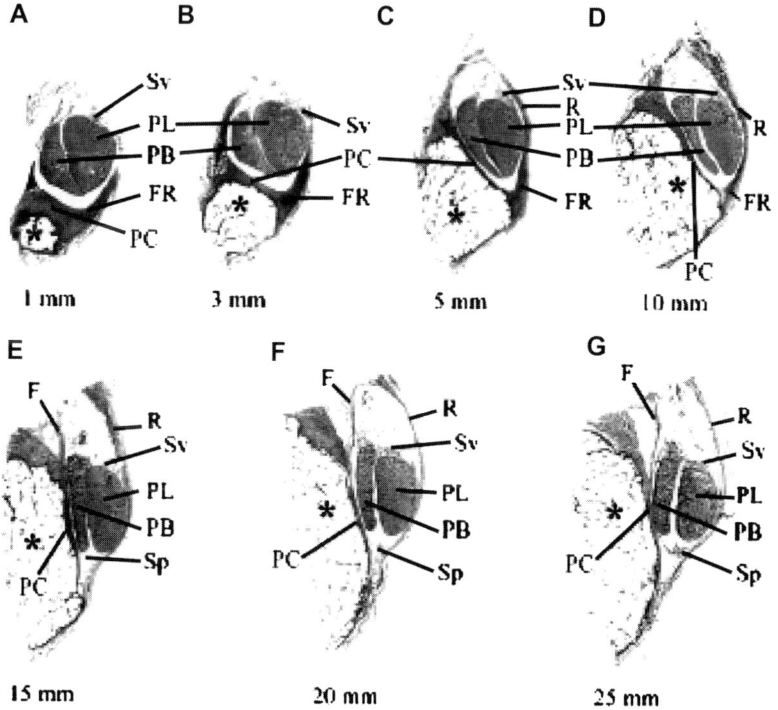

Fig. 2. Serial transverse sections through the malleolar groove and its contained tendons, peroneus brevis (PB) and peroneus longus (PL). The sections are taken at 1, 3, 5, 10, 15, 20 and 25 mm from the tip of the lateral malleolus (*A–G*, respectively). The top of each figure is posterior. At the distal end of the groove (1- and 3-mm sample points), the periosteal cushion (PC) is thick and together with the prominent fibrous ridge (FR) its shape compensates for the convexity of the lateral malleolus (*) in these regions. More proximally (ie at all other sample points), the groove is either flat or slightly concave, and the associated periosteal cushion is thus much less prominent. At all sample points 5 mm or more from the tip of the malleolus, the superior peroneal retinaculum (R) forms much of the lateral border of the groove. The synovial sheath associated with the peroneal tendons is present in all regions, but its parietal layer (Sp) is only visible at the 15- to 25-mm sample points. Although the visceral layer of the sheath (Sv) is present throughout, it is restricted to the sides of the tendons facing away from the bone. All sections are stained with Masson's trichrome. F is a band of fibrous tissue continuous with the purely fibrous periosteum at this proximal part of the malleolar groove. (*From* Kumai T, Benjamin M. The histological structure of the malleolar groove of the fibula in man: its direct bearing on the displacement of peroneal tendons and their surgical repair. J Anat 2003;203(2): 259; with permission.)

described following skiing injuries, when there has been a sudden deceleration causing forced dorsiflexion of the ankle [27,28], but is also described in many other sports, such as soccer, basketball, rugby, cycling, rowing, baseball, and horse riding [2–8]. During the injury, there is a severe contraction of the peroneal muscles, causing subluxation of the tendons, rupture of the SPR or its attachment, and dislocation of the tendons anteriorly [22,23,27,29,30].

Peroneal tendon dislocation occurs most frequently after a forced dorsiflexion injury but has also been noted when the foot has been in a plantarflexed, inverted, everted, or externally rotated position [23,28,30]. It is thought that these positions are associated with this injury because of tightening of the calcaneofibular ligament, which elevates the floor of the tunnel, causing displacement of the tendons while under extreme load [28].

Several anatomical features can predispose the peroneal tendons to dislocation. These features include a shallow peroneal groove, insufficiency or absence of the SPR, calcaneovalgus deformity, subfibula crowding due to a peroneus quartus, and a low-lying peroneus brevis muscle (Fig. 3) [14,19,24,27].

Associated injuries include calcaneal fracture, peroneal tendon tears, lateral ligament disruption, and intra-articular lesions, such as fibrosis, osteochondral lesions, and loose bodies (Fig. 4) [3,8,12,19,29,31].

Congenital dislocation occurs in 3.3% of neonates, with over 90% resolving without treatment. The resistant cases are often associated with hindfoot deformity or neuromuscular disorder [32]. In the adult, nontraumatic dislocations are believed to be due to deficiencies in the SPR, a shallow groove, or a convex distal fibula [10].

Classification

Peroneal tendon dislocation has been classified by Eckert and Davis into three grades [27].

In grade 1 injuries, the dislocated tendons strip the superficial peroneal retinaculum from the lateral fibula, leaving the fibrocartilage rim attached. In grade 2 injuries, the fibrocartilage rim has also been stripped away. In grade 3 injuries, the retinaculum and fibrocartilage rim pull off an avulsion fracture with them.

Diagnosis

The diagnosis of the acute injury can be easily missed and is often confused with an ankle sprain. Both present with a history of a sporting injury, with

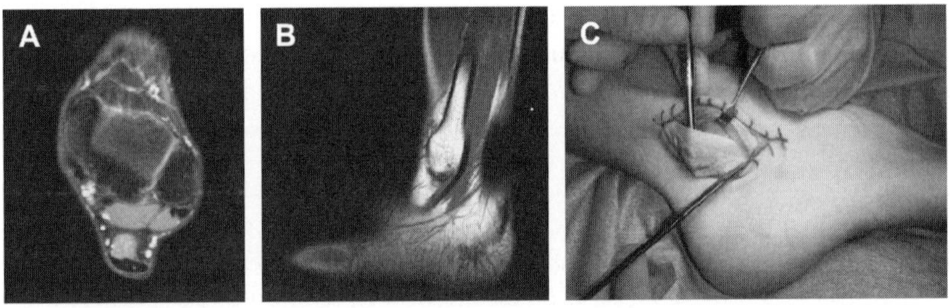

Fig. 3. MRI (*A*, *B*) and intraoperative photograph (*C*) showing a low-lying peroneus brevis, with the muscle belly extending to the level of the ankle joint and below.

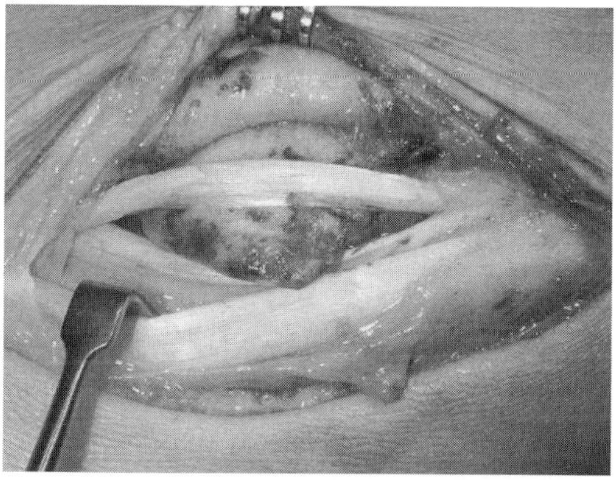

Fig. 4. Acute peroneal dislocation with the peroneus brevis split over the leading edge of the fibular groove. Note the ecchymosis is consistent with an acute dislocation. (*Courtesy of* M. Davies, London.)

swelling, tenderness, and ecchymosis over the lateral aspect of the ankle, and both can occur together [13]. Certain features of the history and examination should alert the clinician to the diagnosis of a peroneal dislocation.

The classic history of an "inversion injury" for a sprain is usually missing, although peroneal dislocation can still occur in plantarflexion, inversion, eversion, or external rotation [23,30]. A peroneal dislocation is more likely with a history of forced dorsiflexion, especially if the ankle is restrained in a ski boot or similar footwear. The maximum area of tenderness and swelling lie posterior to the fibula, rather than anteriorly over the anterior talofibular ligament, and there is significant pain and apprehension, with eversion of the ankle.

In chronic cases, there is often a history of popping or snapping tendons and the dislocated tendons may be visible, lying on top of the fibula. The patient is frequently able to demonstrate the tendons dislocating and there is often a history of instability of the ankle. In the chronic setting, there is little tenderness or swelling and the ligaments are usually intact, with a stable anterior drawer test. The tendons may freely dislocate on activation of the peroneals, with dorsiflexion and eversion (Fig. 5A), and the patient may be able to demonstrate this (Fig. 5B). If the dislocation is not obvious, a guiding digit can help find it (Fig. 5C). The use of a guiding digit is often easier with the patient on his or her side and fully relaxed on an examination couch.

Imaging

Plain radiographs are normal in most cases, but may show an avulsion fracture from the lateral surface of the fibula, consistent with an Eckert grade 3 injury. This fragment may be obscured on an antero-posterior view and thus may only be visible on the mortise view.

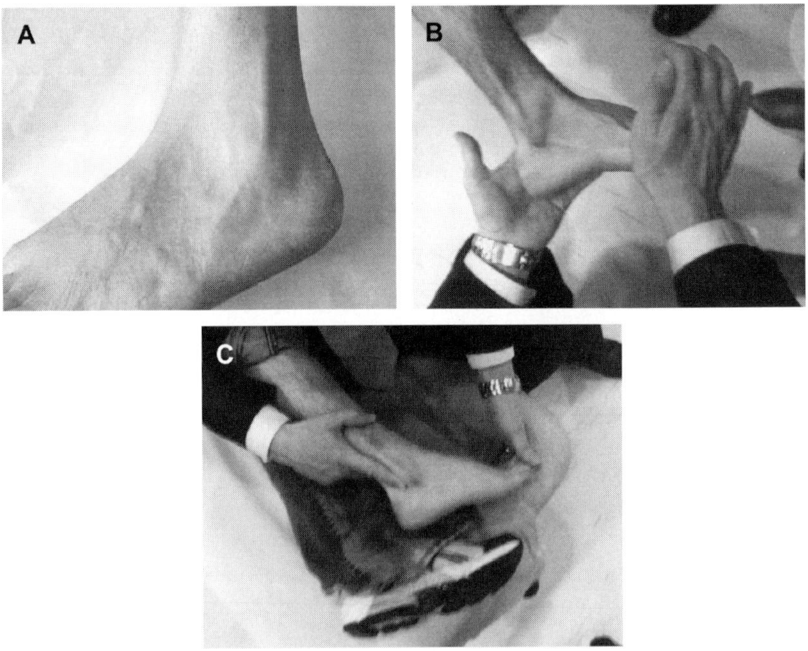

Fig. 5. (*A*) Dislocated peroneal tendons prominent at rest. (*B*) Active dorsiflexion and eversion accentuates dislocation. (*C*) Guiding digit assisting dislocation with the patient lying on side.

CT scanning has been shown to be reliable in diagnosing peroneal dislocation and this is of particular use in the context of calcaneal fractures. Recent advances in software have made CT diagnosis easier with the use of three-dimensional volume-rendered images (Fig. 6) [11,31,33–36].

An MRI scan is the investigation of choice. The scan clearly demonstrates peroneal dislocations and identifies any associated injuries, such as peroneus brevis and longus tears, lateral ligament tears, avulsion fractures, and intra-articular lesions of the ankle joint. The scan also identifies any predisposing causes, such as a convex distal fibula, a low-lying peroneus brevis muscle, or peroneus quartus (Fig. 7A, B).

Treatment

Acute injury

Nonoperative management

Few reports have examined the use of casts, straps, and compression bandages, and most investigators recommend operative repair of an acute injury. The largest study of conservative management, by Escalas and colleagues [12], reported a 74% failure rate in 38 cases after immobilization in compression bandages. A study by Stover and Bryan [28] in 1962 reported

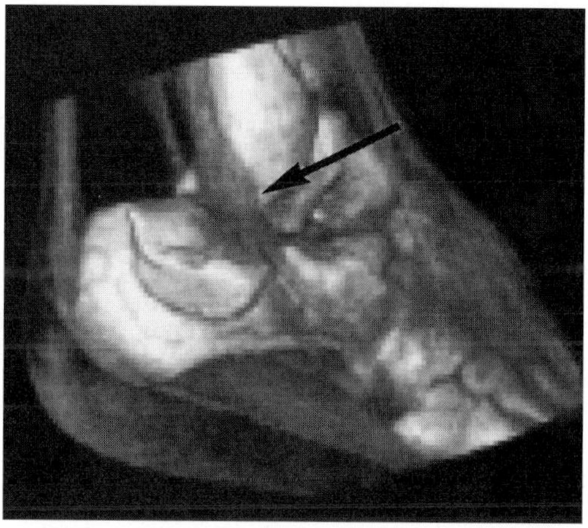

Fig. 6. Three-dimensional volume rendered CT image of ankle. Arrow shows Peroneus Brevis and Longus tendons lying dislocated anteriorly. (*From* Ohashi K, Restrepo JM, El-Khoury GY, et al. Peroneal tendon subluxation and dislocation: detection on volume-rendered images—initial experience. Radiology 2007;242(1):258; with permission.)

on 16 peroneal dislocations treated with either a non–weight-bearing cast for 6 weeks, a weight-bearing cast for 6 weeks, or ankle strapping in neutral. Six out of nine strapped ankles and one weight-bearing cast re-dislocated. None of the five cases treated in a non–weight-bearing cast, in semiequinus, re-dislocated.

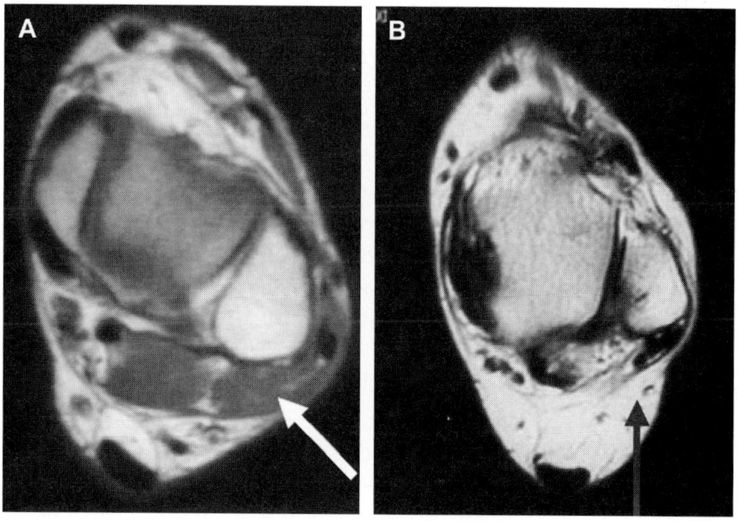

Fig. 7. (*A*) Chronic dislocation of peroneus longus and brevis with low-lying peroneus brevis muscle belly (*arrow*). (*B*) Peroneus quartus tendon causing crowding of the fibular groove (*arrow*).

Operative management

With the patient in the lateral position, a direct repair is performed. Under general, regional or local anesthesia, thigh tourniquet inflated, the posterior aspect of the fibula is exposed through an incision in line with, but a few millimeters behind, the posterior border of the fibula. The incision starts 5 cm above the fibula tip and extends 1 to 2 cm beyond it, in line with the tendons. The sheath is opened longitudinally and extending down as far as the CFL. Anteriorly, the retinaculum is stripped from the fibula forming a pocket, within which the dislocated peroneal tendons may lie. Underneath the dislocated peroneal tendons is a bare area of bleeding fibula. The stripped retinaculum may have the fibrocartilage labrum or an avulsion fragment attached to it. The tendons should be inspected and any tears should be repaired, low-lying muscle bellies resected, and accessory muscles excised. The tendons can then be relocated in the groove and the retinaculum reattached to the fibula with bone sutures or anchors. If there are any large avulsion fragments, these should be fixed back in place. Any smaller fragments can be excised. The sheath is closed without imbrication and the skin closed in layers. Most investigators recommend postoperative immobilization in a cast for 6 weeks. A walker boot can be used after 2 weeks and passive physiotherapy started.

Chronic injury

In chronic cases, surgery is usually necessary because it is rare for this to be asymptomatic. The surgical procedures can be divided into five main categories: (1) SPR reattachment, (2) SPR reconstruction, (3) rerouting procedures, (4) bone block procedures, and (5) groove-deepening procedures.

SPR reattachment

This technique for repairing a chronic injury is the same as that for direct repair described above. The incision of the sheath and exposure of the retinacular pocket are the same. However, in chronic cases, the bare surface of the fibula requires roughening to encourage bleeding and a satisfactory repair. The retinaculum may be attenuated and any excess tissue should be excised before closure. In 1976, Eckert and Davis [27] published a large series of 73 cases treated by SPR reattachment, with only 3 re-dislocations, albeit with a short follow-up of only 6 months. In 1985, Das De and Balasubramaniam [13] likened the stripped retinacular pocket to the Bankart lesion of the shoulder and reported on a direct repair, termed the Singapore operation, using sutures to reattach the SPR to the fibula and termed it the Singapore operation. In 1998, Hui and colleagues [16] reported on the long-term results of 21 cases at 9.3 years. There were no recurrences and 18 out of 21 patients had good or excellent results. A more recent publication by Adachi and colleagues [5] in 2006 presents the results of 18 cases of SPR reattachment using a tissue tensioner device to achieve a specified retinacular tension. At 2 years, all had returned to their preinjury level of activity with no recurrences and an average American Orthopaedic Foot & Ankle Society (AOFAS) score of 93 (Fig. 8).

SPR reconstruction

Reconstruction of the SPR using both local and free grafts has been described. In 1932, Jones [37] published a technique using a strip of the lateral Achilles to reconstruct the posterior band of the SPR. With this technique, a small strip of the lateral Achilles tendon is harvested, leaving the base attached to the calcaneum. The strip must have adequate length to reach the distal fibula and is attached via a drill hole. The repair must be performed with the foot in full dorsiflexion to prevent over-tightening. Otherwise, a tenodesis will occur blocking full dorsiflexion. In 1980, Escalas and colleagues [12] reported on 15 cases using this procedure. At 6.8 years, 14 were asymptomatic and had returned to full activity. One patient had symptoms of insecurity of the ankle but with no clinical signs of instability. Other grafts have been used to augment the SPR, including the plantaris tendon [4] and a gracilis graft (Fig. 9) [17].

Rerouting procedures

This technique employs the CFL as a soft tissue restraint to further dislocation of the peroneal tendons. To accomplish this, either (1) the peroneal tendons are transferred beneath the CFL by division of the tendons or (2) the CFL is detached and transferred over the tendons. Poll and Duijfjes

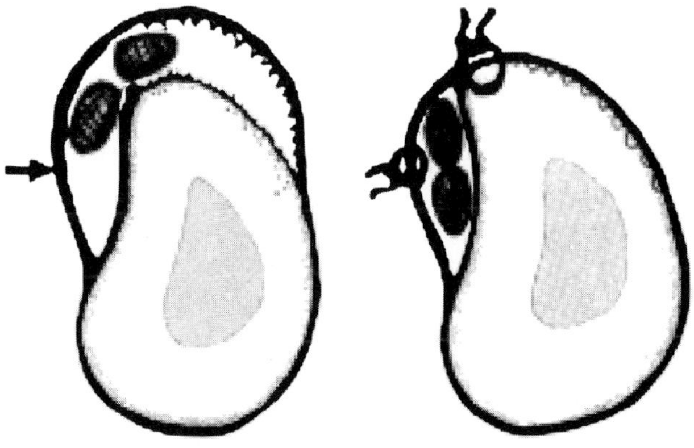

Fig. 8. Diagrams of transverse sections of the lower end of the left fibula seen from above. (*Left figure*) The false pouch formed by stripping of periosteum from the lateral malleolus in continuity with the superior peroneal retinaculum. The arrow shows the site for incision of the retinaculum. (*Right figure*) Normal anatomy is restored by obliteration of the false pouch and closing the incision in the peroneal retinaculum. (*From* Das De S, Balasubramaniam P. A repair operation for recurrent dislocation of peroneal tendons. J Bone Joint Surg Br 1985;67(4):585; with permission.)

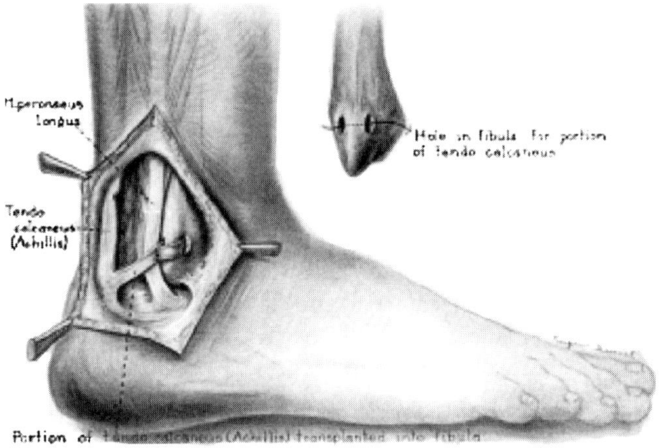

Fig. 9. The Jones operation. (*From* Jones E. Operative treatment of chronic dislocation of the peroneal tendons. J Bone and Joint Surg 1932;14:575; with permission.)

[14] describe a technique of CFL transfer on an inferiorly based bone block from the calcaneum and subsequent fixation. They report on 10 ankles with an average follow-up of 4 years, with no recurrences and 9 out of 10 returning to their preinjury sports. Two patients complained of slight pain, 3 of swelling, and 4 of reduced sensation around the scar. Pozo and Jackson [21] describe a similar technique with proximal detachment of the CFL on a fibula bone block.

In 1975, Sarmiento and Wolf [23] described division of the peroneal tendons and rerouting them beneath the CFL. In 1986, Martens [22] published the results of over 11 cases at 30 months with no recurrences and all patients continuing at previous activity levels but again with 1 patient complaining of pain and swelling, another with stiffness, and 2 with sural nerve injury. Platzgummer first described division of the CFL and repair over the peroneal tendons in 1967. The results in 13 cases were reviewed by Steinbock and Pinsger [15] with 11 excellent results and 2 results, with occasional pain and swelling, graded good (Fig. 10).

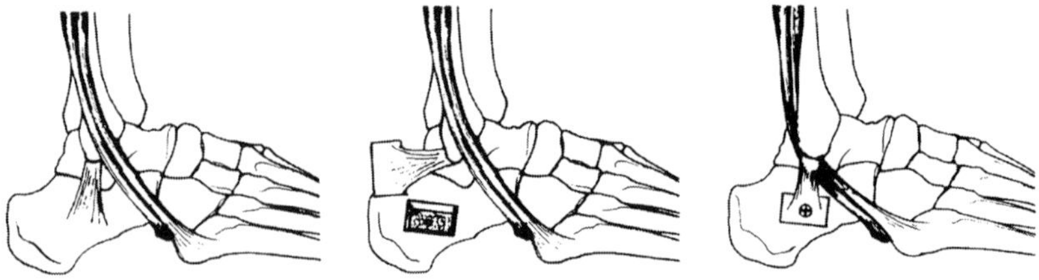

Fig. 10. (*From* Poll RG, Duijfjes F. The treatment of recurrent dislocation of the peroneal tendons. J Bone Joint Surg Br 1984;66(1):99; with permission.)

Groove-deepening procedures

There are several published methods for deepening the fibula groove, all combined with a direct repair of the SPR. The main principle of the procedure is to depress the floor of the groove further to accentuate it and prevent re-dislocation. A variety of techniques have been used [29]. Zoellner and Clancy [20] describe a simple technique of deepening the groove by local excision of bone and excavation. Twelve consecutive cases are reviewed by Kollias and Ferkel [3] at 8 months with no recurrences, and 91% returning to full activity. Karlsson and colleagues [2] presents the results after 3.5 years on 15 patients treated by deepening the groove with a curved chisel and repair of the retinaculum. There were no recurrences and good or excellent results in 87% of cases with 13% fair due to postoperative stiffness and pain on exertion. In 2005, Porter and colleagues [6] described a modification of this technique with recession of the posterior cortex and repair of the SPR. Rather than employing standard postoperative cast immobilization, a walker boot was used with physiotherapy starting at 1 week postsurgery. Fourteen ankles were followed up for 3 years with no recurrences, minimal postoperative symptoms, and an average return to sports of 3 months.

Bone block procedures

The principle of bone block procedures is to accentuate the outer wall of the groove and increase the bony restraint to dislocation. Kelly first described this in 1920 [7], using a distal fibula bone block, which is displaced

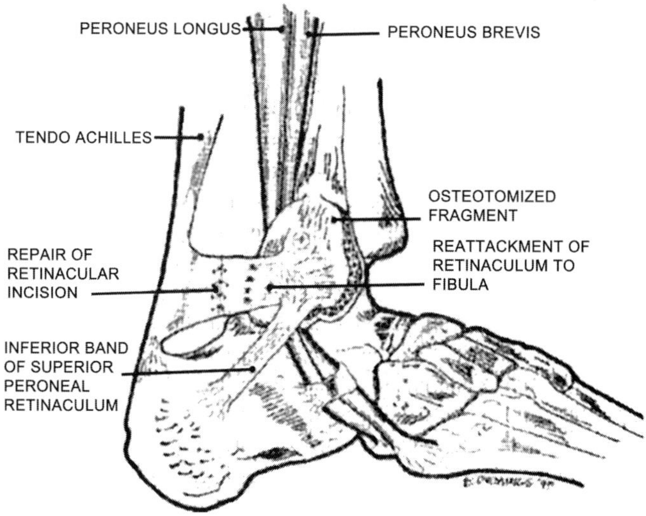

Fig. 11. Diagram shows a bone block procedure to deepen the fibula groove using a rotational osteotomy of the outer half of distal fibula. (*From* Mason RB, Henderson JP. Traumatic peroneal tendon instability. Am J Sports Med 1996;24(5):656; with permission.)

posteriorly and internally fixed. Mason and Henderson [8] reported on this technique in 1996. They describe a rotational osteotomy of the distal fibula, which deepens the groove by accentuating the bony lateral wall (Fig. 11). There were five acute and six chronic dislocations treated with a rotational osteotomy of the distal fibula [8]. At 29 months, nine cases had an excellent result with one re-dislocation and one case of recurrent osteomyelitis with the fibula osteotomy forming a sequestrum. Two patients complained of mild pain over prominent screws, there was one case of sural nerve injury, and all patients returned to their previous levels of activity.

There are several variations of the bone block technique, including the Duvries posterior sliding graft and inferior sliding grafts using a bone block to augment the groove distally [18]. Larsen [24] reports a significant number of complications using the Duvries method with a 22% complication rate due to screw malposition, malleolar fractures, or graft fractures. The results were unsatisfactory in 14% because of re-dislocation, subluxation, or instability.

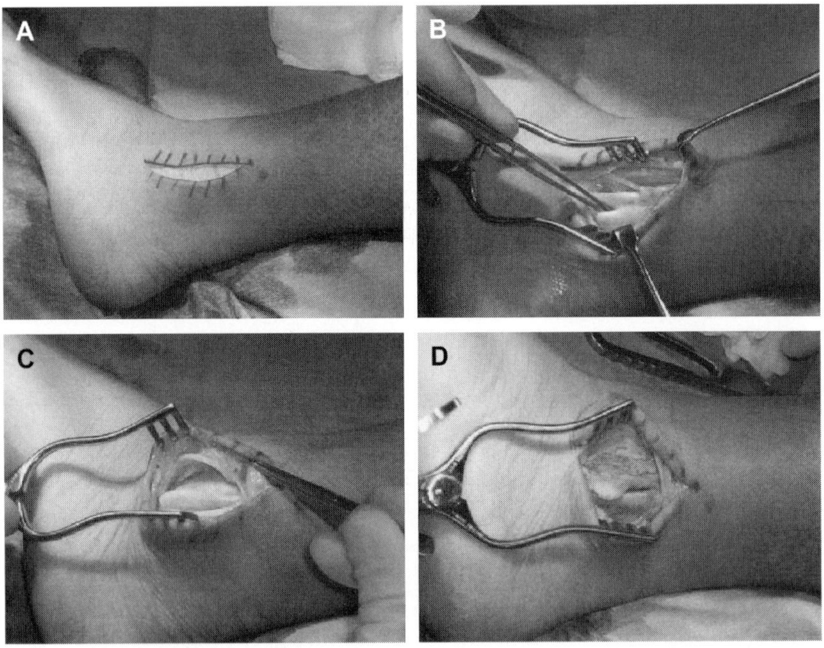

Fig. 12. (*A*) The incision to repair a peroneal tendon dislocation is in line with the posterior border of the fibula for approximately 5 cm to the tip. Care is taken to avoid the sural nerve, which follows a similar course approximately 1 cm posteriorly. (*B*) In repairing a peroneal tendon dislocation, the sheath is opened in line with the skin incision. In this case, a split of the peroneus brevis lies either side of the fibrocartilage edge. (*C*) Another view of opening during repair of peroneal tendon dislocation. (*D*) Another view of opening during repair of peroneal tendon dislocation.

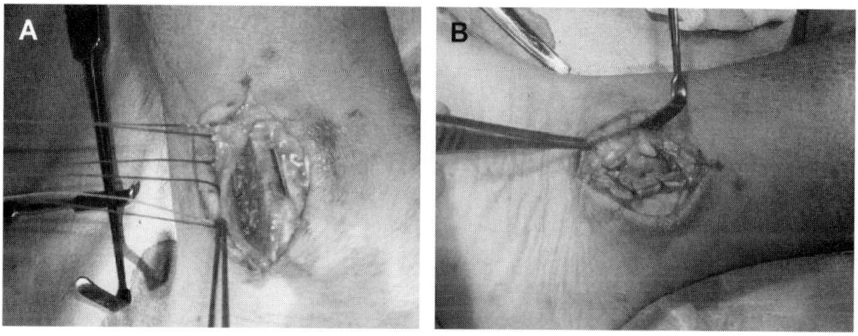

Fig. 13. (*A*) In repairing a peroneal tendon dislocation, the retinaculum is reattached using bone sutures and the sheath closed after resection of any lax tissue. (*B*) Another view of reattachment of retinaculum using bone sutures during repair of peroneal tendon dislocation. The sheath closed after resection of any lax tissue.

Author's preferred treatment

For the acute or chronic injury, the author recommends the direct repair described above. If there is any concern regarding instability, then the author performs a groove-deepening procedure using a burr. The periosteum and fibrocartilage covering the floor of the groove is elevated by sharp dissection and the groove deepened by 3 to 4 mm with a burr. The periosteal/fibrocartilage layer is replaced afterwards and sutured (Fig. 12A–D).

After reduction of the tendons, the anterior pocket of a chronic tear is evident. The bare area of fibula is roughened to encourage bleeding and scarring (Note: The fibrocartilage is not torn—grade 1 injury) (Fig. 13A, B).

Postoperative management

The ankle is placed in a below-knee, non–weight-bearing temporary cast, in semiequinus for 2 weeks. This is changed to a walker boot, fully weight-bearing, for 4 weeks and passive physiotherapy started. At the 6-week stage, the patient can mobilize fully weight-bearing out of the walker boot and a full active physiotherapy program is started, with an expected return to sports of between 4 and 6 months.

Summary

Peroneal tendon dislocation is an infrequent sports injury and can be difficult to diagnose. Posterior fibula tenderness and pain with eversion are useful signs to discriminate this from an ankle sprain. In the acute setting, a direct repair provides good results but may need to be augmented with additional soft tissue or bony restraints. For chronic injuries, there are several methods of reconstruction, all with acceptable outcomes, although bone block procedures have the highest rate of secondary procedures.

References

[1] Monteggia GB. Instituzini Chirurgiche. Parte Secondu. Milan; 1803. p. 336–41.

[2] Karlsson J, Eriksson BI, Sward L. Recurrent dislocation of the peroneal tendons. Scand J Med Sci Sports 1996;6(4):242–6.

[3] Kollias SL, Ferkel RD. Fibular grooving for recurrent peroneal tendon subluxation. Am J Sports Med 1997;25(3):329–35.

[4] Hansen BH. Reconstruction of the peroneal retinaculum using the plantaris tendon: a case report. Scand J Med Sci Sports 1996;6(6):355–8.

[5] Adachi N, Fukuhara K, Tanaka H, et al. Superior retinaculoplasty for recurrent dislocation of peroneal tendons. Foot Ankle Int 2006;27(12):1074–8.

[6] Porter D, McCarroll J, Knapp E, et al. Peroneal tendon subluxation in athletes: fibular groove deepening and retinacular reconstruction. Foot Ankle Int 2005;26(6):436–41.

[7] Kelly RE. An operation for the chronic dislocation of the peroneal tendons. Br J Surg 1920;7: 502–4.

[8] Mason RB, Henderson JP. Traumatic peroneal tendon instability. Am J Sports Med 1996; 24(5):652–8.

[9] Clanton Thomas O. Athletic injuries to the soft tissues of the foot and ankle. In: Coughlin MJ, Mann RA, editors. Surgery of the foot and ankle. 7th edition. St. Louis (MO): Mosby; 1999.

[10] Frey CC, Shereff MJ. Tendon injuries about the ankle in athletes. Clin Sports Med 1988;7(1): 103–18.

[11] Ebraheim NA, Zeiss J, Skie MC, et al. Radiological evaluation of peroneal tendon pathology associated with calcaneal fractures. J Orthop Trauma 1991;5(3):365–9.

[12] Escalas F, Figueras JM, Merino JA. Dislocation of the peroneal tendons. Long-term results of surgical treatment. J Bone Joint Surg Am 1980;62(3):451–3.

[13] Das De S, Balasubramaniam P. A repair operation for recurrent dislocation of peroneal tendons. J Bone Joint Surg Br 1985;67(4):585–7.

[14] Poll RG, Duijfjes F. The treatment of recurrent dislocation of the peroneal tendons. J Bone Joint Surg Br 1984;66(1):98–100.

[15] Steinbock G, Pinsger M. Treatment of peroneal tendon dislocation by transposition under the calcaneofibular ligament. Foot Ankle Int 1994;15(3):107–11.

[16] Hui JH, Das De S, Balasubramaniam P. The Singapore operation for recurrent dislocation of peroneal tendons: long-term results. J Bone Joint Surg Br 1998;80(2):325–7.

[17] Miyamoto W, Takao M, Komatu F, et al. Reconstruction of the superior peroneal retinaculum using an autologous gracilis tendon graft for chronic dislocation of the peroneal tendons accompanied by lateral instability of the ankle: technical note. Knee Surg Sports Traumatol Arthrosc 2007;15(4):461–4, Epub 2006 Dec 23.

[18] Micheli LJ, Waters PM, Sanders DP. Sliding fibular graft repair for chronic dislocation of the peroneal tendons. Am J Sports Med 1989;17(1):68–71.

[19] Mendicino RW, Orsini RC, Whitman SE, et al. Fibular groove deepening for recurrent peroneal subluxation. J Foot Ankle Surg 2001;40(4):252–63.

[20] Zoellner G, Clancy W Jr. Recurrent dislocation of the peroneal tendon. J Bone Joint Surg Am 1979;61(2):292–4.

[21] Pozo JL, Jackson AM. A rerouting operation for dislocation of peroneal tendons: operative technique and case report. Foot Ankle 1984;5(1):42–4.

[22] Martens MA, Noyez JF, Mulier JC. Recurrent dislocation of the peroneal tendons. Results of rerouting the tendons under the calcaneofibular ligament. Am J Sports Med 1986;14(2): 148–50.

[23] Sarmiento A, Wolf M. Subluxation of peroneal tendons. Case treated by rerouting tendons under calcaneofibular ligament. J Bone Joint Surg Am 1975;57(1):115–6.

[24] Larsen E, Flink-Olsen M, Seerup K. Surgery for recurrent dislocation of the peroneal tendons. Acta Orthop Scand 1984;55(5):554–5.

[25] Kumai T, Benjamin M. The histological structure of the malleolar groove of the fibula in man: its direct bearing on the displacement of peroneal tendons and their surgical repair. J Anat 2003;203(2):257–62.

[26] Edwards ME. The relationship of the peroneal tendons to the fibula, calcaneus and cuboideum. Am J Anat 1928;42:213–53.

[27] Eckert WR, Davis EA Jr. Acute rupture of the peroneal retinaculum. J Bone Joint Surg Am 1976;58(5):670–2.

[28] Stover CN, Bryan DR. Traumatic dislocation of the peroneal tendons. Am J Surg 1962;103: 180–6.

[29] Arrowsmith SR, Fleming LL, Allman FL. Traumatic dislocations of the peroneal tendons. Am J Sports Med 1983;11(3):142–6.

[30] Marti R. Dislocation of the peroneal tendons. Am J Sports Med 1977;5(1):19–22.

[31] Bradley SA, Davies AM. Computed tomographic assessment of soft tissue abnormalities following calcaneal fractures. Br J Radiol 1992;65:105–11.

[32] Purnell ML, Drummond DS, Engber WD, et al. Congenital dislocation of the peroneal tendons in the calcaneovalgus foot. J Bone Joint Surg Br 1983;65(3):316–9.

[33] Rosenberg ZS, Feldman F, Singson RD, et al. Peroneal tendon injury associated with calcaneal fractures: CT findings. Am J Roentgenol 1987;149:125–9.

[34] Rosenberg ZS, Feldman F, Singson RD. Peroneal tendon injuries: CT analysis. Radiology 1986;161:743–8.

[35] Ho RT, Smith D, Escobedo E. Peroneal tendon dislocation: CT diagnosis and clinical importance. AJR Am J Roentgenol 2001;177:1193.

[36] Ohashi K, Restrepo JM, El-Khoury GY, et al. Peroneal tendon subluxation and dislocation: detection on volume-rendered images—initial experience. Radiology 2007;242(1):252–7.

[37] Jones E. Operative treatment of chronic dislocation of the peroneal tendons. J Bone and Joint Surg 1932;14:574–6.

ELSEVIER
SAUNDERS

Foot Ankle Clin N Am
12 (2007) 659–674

FOOT AND
ANKLE CLINICS

Acute Peroneal Tendon Tears

H.K. Slater, MB, BS, FRACS, FAOrthA

North Sydney Orthopaedic and Sports Medicine Centre, 286 Pacific Highway, Crows Nest, NSW 2065, Sydney, Australia

Acute peroneal tendon tears present as a relatively sudden onset of lateral ankle or hindfoot pain, frequently in conjunction with a traumatic episode or injury. Underlying or causative factors, including recurrent ankle sprains, hindfoot varus leading to ankle instability, or dislocating peroneal tendons may be associated and can often lead to peroneal tendon tears being overlooked as a cause of persistent lateral ankle or foot pain. Some apparently acute peroneal tendon tears may represent an acute manifestation of an underlying chronic or subclinical abnormality.

The spectrum of peroneal tendinopathies includes tenosynovitis, tendinosis, subluxation or dislocation, stenosing tenosynovitis, disorders of the os peroneum, and conditions related to accessory peroneal tendons, as well as acute and chronic tendon tears. These abnormalities of the peroneal tendons may coexist, and one may lead to another, as evidenced by the significant incidence of tears in the presence of dislocating peronei and ankle instability.

Suspicion of the possibility of peroneal tendon injury, coupled with careful clinical examination and appropriate investigation, allows the clinician to identify the extent of damage and to implement a successful management plan. Because peroneal tears signify a mechanical abnormality, this management often entails surgical intervention.

Anatomy and biomechanics

The peroneal muscles constitute the lateral compartment of the lower leg. The peroneus brevis arises from the mid-third of the fibula and has a low-lying muscle belly extending almost to the level of the ankle joint. At this level, it has a flattened ovoid shape as it passes posterior to the distal fibular shaft, where it articulates with and glides on a fibrocartilage lining within the

E-mail address: hks1@optusnet.com.au

1083-7515/07/$ - see front matter
doi:10.1016/j.fcl.2007.07.008

retromalleolar groove. The peroneus longus arises more proximally from both tibia and fibula, and forms a rounded tendon, which lies immediately posterior to the peroneus brevis as it approaches the tip of the fibula. The superior peroneal retinaculum arises from the posterolateral aspect of the distal fibula to act as a restraint to enclose the peroneal tendons in a common sheath, which extends to just below the fibular tip, where each tendon begins to occupy a separate sheath. The peroneus longus now passes inferior to the peroneal tubercle, thence into the cuboid tunnel, and obliquely across the undersurface of the midfoot to attach predominantly to the base of the first metatarsal and medial cuneiform. Thus, the peroneus longus acts as a plantar flexor of the ankle and foot, an evertor of the foot, and a plantar flexor of the first metatarsal. The os peroneum is a sesamoid bone lying within the tendon of peroneus longus as it passes under the cuboid. It is thought to be present in 10% to 20% of the population, and can be a source of pain, leading to rupture of the peroneus longus in some cases.

The peroneus brevis passes superior to the peroneal tubercle and attaches to the base of the fifth metatarsal at the styloid process. The peroneus brevis thus acts as a plantar flexor of the ankle and foot, and as an evertor of the foot. These dynamic stabilizers of the lateral aspect of the ankle provide an important function in resisting inversion and in acting as antagonists of the medial tendons, including the tibialis posterior [1].

The superior peroneal retinaculum, because it has a strong fibrous attachment to the posterolateral aspect of the fibula, is the main restraint preventing subluxation or dislocation of the peronei around the tip of the fibula [2]. The depth of the fibular groove is also a factor [3]. A deep groove makes the peroneal tendon less prone to dislocation, while a shallow groove, by allowing the peronei to more readily stress the fibrous attachment of the superior peroneal retinaculum, occasionally leads to disruption of the attachment and peroneal tendon dislocation (Fig. 1) [4]. The inferior peroneal

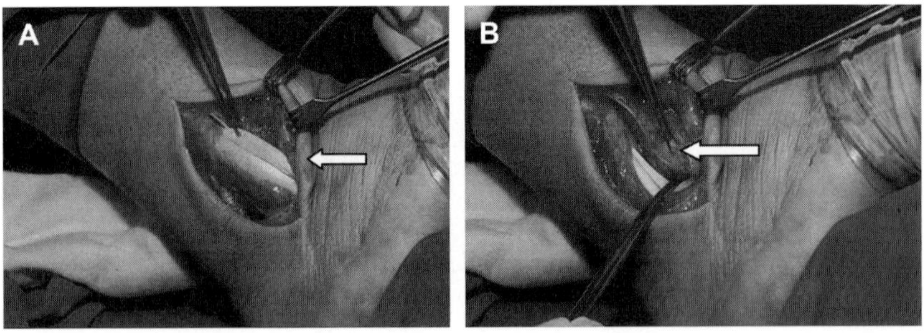

Fig. 1. (*A*) Dislocation of both peroneal tendons, with tendons (*arrow*) lying lateral to the tip of the fibula. Recurrent dislocation causes mechanical irritation of the peronei and eventual tears may occur. (*B*) With the peronei reduced, a fibro-periosteal flap (*arrow*) can be seen at the tip of the fibula. This flap should be incorporated into the repair of the superior peroneal retinaculum.

retinaculum blends with the thickened sheath of both tendons at the level of the peroneal tubercle.

The peroneus quartus is an accessory peroneal tendon reported to occur in 13% to 22% of the population [5,6]. It inserts into the lateral wall of the calcaneus and may be associated with an enlarged peroneal tubercle, thus predisposing to stenosing tenosynovitis. Anatomic variants should be considered when assessing the possibility of peroneal tendon tears [7].

A cadaver study by Petersen and colleagues [8] suggests that there are three relatively avascular zones within the peronei, and these zones correspond to the locations of most peroneal tendon tears. Both the peroneus longus and brevis have reduced vascularity adjacent to the tip of the fibula, a common site for tears, particularly in the peroneus brevis (Fig. 2) [9]. The peroneus longus also has reduced vascularity at the cuboid tunnel, where rupture may occur in association with an os peroneum [10,11].

The peroneus longus provides 35% and the peroneus brevis 28% of hindfoot eversion power [12]. Together, the peroneus longus and brevis contribute only 4% of ankle plantarflexion power, the majority being provided by the gastrocnemius and soleus muscles.

A neutral hindfoot on weight-bearing allows for balanced ankle motors, without additional stress on the peronei. Hindfoot varus due to pes cavus leads to increased stress in the peronei, predisposing to tenosynovitis [13]. Similarly, lateral ankle instability with recurrent inversion episodes leads to microtrauma to the peronei and eventual macroscopic tears [9,14–21]. Tears are also seen in the valgus arthritic ankle as the tendons become

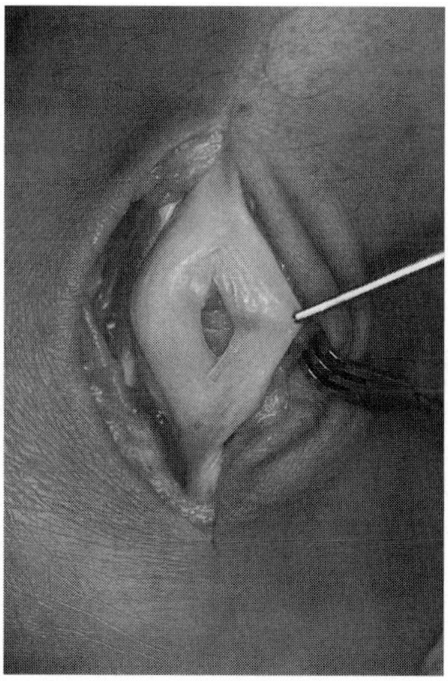

Fig. 2. The most common peroneal tear is in the form of a "buttonhole" tear of the peroneus brevis at the level of the tip of the fibula.

crowded in the retromalleolar space and the subfibular recess. These tears tend to be chronic rather than acute and are discussed elsewhere in this issue (Fig. 3).

Etiology of peroneal tendon tears

Anatomic variants may predispose to peroneal tendon tears. Such variants include generalized ligamentous laxity syndromes, which allow subluxation or dislocation and subsequent tearing of the peronei. A shallow retromalleolar groove also predisposes to subluxation and dislocation [3]. Ankles with recurrent instability or arthrosis occasionally show ulceration of the fibrocartilage lining of the distal fibula, eventual osteophyte formation with direct abrasion of peroneus brevis over the osteophyte, and resultant splitting. It is likely that a combination of factors cause peroneal tendon tears, including microvascular, mechanical, and anatomical factors [15,16,22–27].

There is a logical mechanical explanation for the incidence of splitting tears in the peroneus brevis in the presence of dislocating peroneal tendons. The flattened peroneus brevis tendon slides over the sharp posterolateral aspect of the fibula after avulsion of the superior peroneal retinaculum attachment, entering a false synovial pouch. Rarely, a flake of bone is avulsed, giving a pathognomonic radiological appearance [28]. Repeated subluxation or dislocation during activity puts great stress on the tendon while under load, causing a fraying effect as the tendons pass under tension around

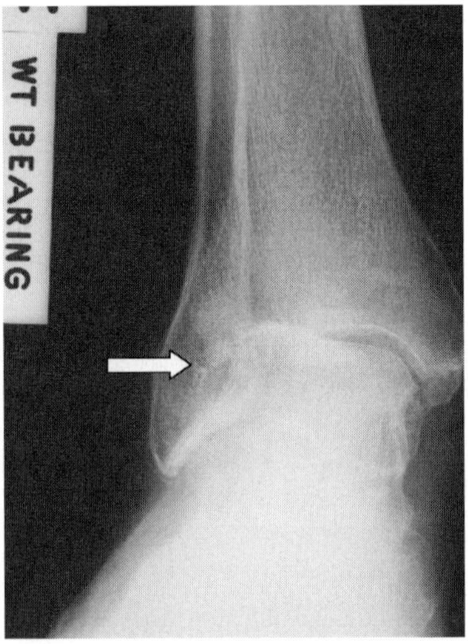

Fig. 3. Weight-bearing radiograph showing valgus erosion (*arrow*), which causes compression of the peronei in the subfibular region and may result in tearing of the tendons.

the tip of the fibula. This magnifies the compressive forces on the tendon, resulting in longitudinal splitting and tearing. If this occurs during vigorous activity, the result may be an acute presentation of a peroneal tear in combination with a peroneal tendon dislocation (Fig. 4) [16].

The incidence of peroneus brevis tears in the presence of lateral ankle instability or a varus hindfoot is thought to be due to repeated compressive forces as the peroneus longus loads the central aspect of the peroneus brevis in the retromalleolar groove, resulting in a longitudinal split, which is bathed in synovial fluid. Because of the relative avascularity, the tear may propagate [16,18,22,27]. This compressive mechanism is not usually associated with subluxation or dislocation of the peronei. Krause and Brodsky [16], however, suggest that subluxation of the peronei is the main cause of peroneus brevis tears.

Clinical presentation

Acute peroneal tendon tears may present following an injury to a previously asymptomatic ankle, or may be identified during imaging or surgery for associated foot and ankle pathology [29,30]. If symptomatic and occurring as a result of injury, the patient may complain of pain located on the lateral aspect of the foot or ankle. Swelling is almost always evident if an underlying peroneal tendon tear is present [16]. Observation of standing hindfoot alignment will alert the clinician to increased hindfoot varus or valgus due to ankle arthrosis, or varus due to pes cavus.

If located adjacent to the tip of the fibula, one or both tendons may be involved, with the peroneus brevis being more commonly injured [22]. Tenderness and swelling more distally, adjacent to the base of the fifth

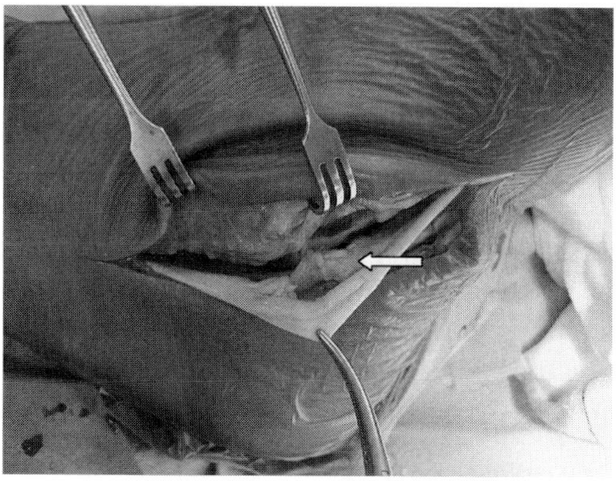

Fig. 4. A ragged "buttonhole" tear in the peroneus brevis, secondary to recurrent peroneal tendon dislocation. Note the ulcerated false synovial pouch (*arrow*) under the distal fibular periosteum.

metatarsal is more likely to indicate damage to the peroneus longus (Fig. 5). The patient who has suffered a dislocation of the peronei usually has swelling and tenderness proximal to the tip of the fibula, and gentle resisted eversion often reproduces the dislocation. This is generally followed by a withdrawal reaction and rapid spontaneous reduction. Depending on the extent of tearing of the superior peroneal retinaculum, dislocation may be demonstrated with resisted eversion in plantarflexion, but sometimes it can only be demonstrated in dorsiflexion. Swelling usually extends above the tip of the fibula and, in the case of complete rupture of one or both tendons, bruising may be evident.

Weakness of the respective tendons can be demonstrated with reduced power of eversion. With peroneus longus injury, there may be reduced power of plantarflexion of the first ray when compared with the normal side. However, these features are not always reliable when there is inhibition due to pain.

Lacerations or puncture wounds on the lateral aspect of the foot should always be considered a potential cause of acute peroneal tendon injury. Broken glass from a falling bottle, for example, can cleanly and completely sever one or both tendons through a small wound if the tendons are under tension (Fig. 6).

In the presence of an acute lateral ankle ligament sprain or a recurrent sprain, tenderness posterior to the distal fibula should raise suspicion of peroneal tendon pathology [16,31]. In the recurrently sprained ankle, an effusion can often be demonstrated in the peroneal sheath if there is an underlying tendon tear. Tears can also be associated with ganglionic in-substance degeneration, and a localized tender nodule in the line of the peroneal tendons may be seen or felt. Such tearing tends to occur adjacent to the peroneal tubercle, which may be enlarged and tender to palpation [32].

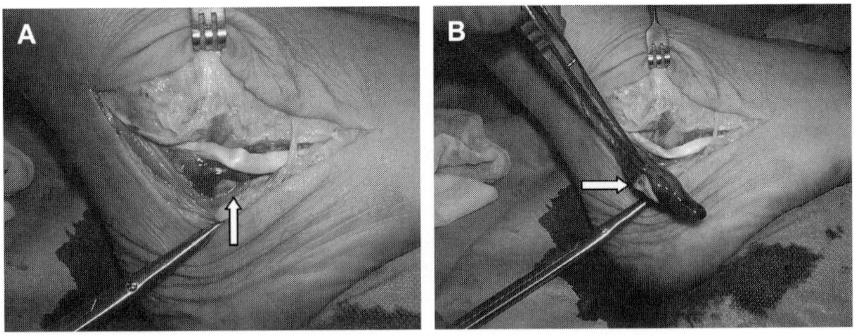

Fig. 5. (*A*) Complete rupture of the peroneus longus, with the hemorrhagic rounded end (*arrow*) of the tendon visible. Note the sural nerve passing obliquely across the distal aspect of the wound. (*B*) White fibrocartilage (*arrow*) of an os peroneum proximal to the peroneus longus rupture.

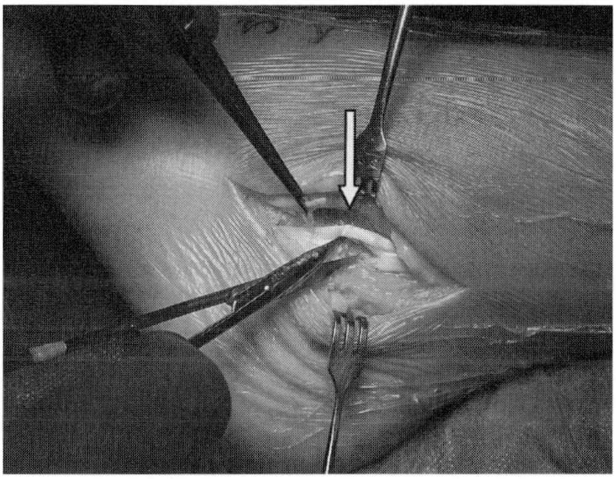

Fig. 6. A central laceration of the peroneus longus (*downward arrow*) in a young woman who suffered a puncture wound by a stingray barb. Despite a 5-mm entry wound, she presented 5 weeks later describing a "snap" while running. Deeper and just distal, the attenuated end of the ruptured peroneus brevis is shown held by forceps.

Os peroneum syndrome [33] may be associated with peroneus longus tears. However, rupture usually occurs distal to the os peroneum.

Investigations

Plain radiography is indicated for the initial assessment of a significant ankle injury as well as for the assessment of lateral ankle pain. Careful observation may show a "flake sign" at the outer aspect of the tip of the fibula, indicating avulsion of the superior peroneal retinaculum [28]. This sign is rarely present, but pathognomonic. In cases of trauma, non–weight-bearing radiographs are performed, but in cases of lateral ankle pain without trauma, weight-bearing radiographs of the foot and ankle provide significantly more information about foot and ankle function. Foot shape, planus or cavus, can be ascertained on weight-bearing radiographs, and sesamoid bones, such as the os peroneum, can be identified. A proximally displaced or fragmented os peroneum is an indicator of peroneus longus disruption [10,11,34,35]. Plain radiographs are not reliable for assessing the size of the peroneal tubercle, although it may be visible in profile on some views.

In the hands of an experienced operator, real-time duplex ultrasonography is an extremely useful tool for the assessment of peroneal tendon pathology [4,36]. It has a high sensitivity and specificity for identifying tenosynovitis and tears of both tendons. It has the advantages of being less expensive and more readily available than MRI scanning, although it is operator-dependent and does not provide as much information as an MRI about adjacent anatomical structures that may also be injured or damaged.

Ultrasonography can demonstrate the fine microarchitecture of the tendons and peritendinous tissues, and provides a rapid and sensitive comparison with the contralateral side. Whereas MRI scanning is a static study, ultrasonography is a dynamic study, which can allow the operator to examine tendon stability and tendon adhesion, and has the advantage of allowing ultrasound-guided injection if indicated. Because of the angled longitudinal course of the tendons, which may create angle artifact on images, MRI is less sensitive and specific for tendonitis. Thus, specific sequences may be required to adequately image the tendons.

Ultrasonography is only superior to MRI scanning, however, if adequate operator expertise is available. If such expertise is unavailable, MRI should be the preferred investigation [29,30,37–42].

Before the availability of reliable ultrasonography and MRI scanning, peroneal tenography was used to image the tendons. However, this invasive modality is now rarely employed.

Some peroneal tears may become evident during the investigation of other ankle disorders or during surgery. Rarely, the peroneal tendons may be visualized during ankle arthroscopy in the presence of severe lateral ankle ligament disruption (Fig. 7).

Management

Factors to consider when planning management of acute peroneal tendon tears include the age of the patient and his or her physical demands, which tendon is involved, and whether there is associated or causative pathology requiring attention. The site of tendon tearing also dictates the preferred method of treatment, as do the quality of the remaining tendon tissue, the extent of tearing, and the viability and excursion of the respective proximal

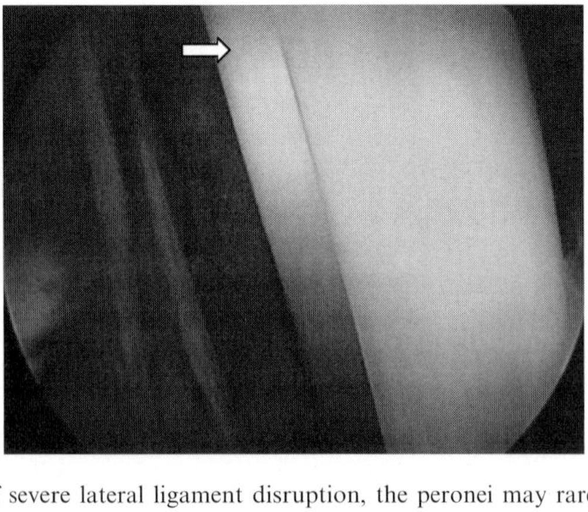

Fig. 7. In cases of severe lateral ligament disruption, the peronei may rarely be seen arthroscopically. In this case, they appear normal (*arrow*).

musculature. Krause and Brodsky [16] classified peroneal tendon tears based on the percentage of viable tendon remaining after debridement, indicating that repair was preferred if 50% or more of the tendon remained after debridement, but tenodesis or tendon transfer if less than 50% of the tendon remained after debridement.

When nonoperative treatment is considered unsuitable, surgical options include direct tendon repair, debridement and tenoplasty, tendon transfer procedures, autogenous soft tissue reconstructions, and tenodesis procedures. During any surgical approach to the lateral aspect of the ankle, the variable anatomy of the sural nerve should be borne in mind so the nerve is properly identified and protected.

An algorithm for the surgical treatment of peroneal tendon tears has been proposed by Redfern and Myerson [22] who stress the importance of residual function in the torn tendons, excursion of the proximal musculature, and the need to consider associated hindfoot deformity and ankle instability.

While peroneal tendoscopy may be used to investigate lateral ankle pain, its place in the presence of ultrasound- or MRI-confirmed peroneal tears remains controversial. As Scholten and van Dijk [43] point out, "miniopen" repair is still required [44].

If peroneus brevis has a longitudinal split or "buttonhole" tear at the tip of the fibula, but there is no transverse defect, either the lateral limb of the torn tendon can be excised in an oblique fashion, or suturing of the defect can be performed (Fig. 8). Suturing relies on the premise that satisfactory healing will occur in tendon tissue that is already abnormal and often swollen. Synovial fluid may delay or prevent healing of the defect. Use of peroneus brevis tendon tissue as an autogenous graft in tenodesis procedures for ankle instability remains an accepted technique [45,46] without significant adverse effects on peroneal function. Therefore excision of the abnormal

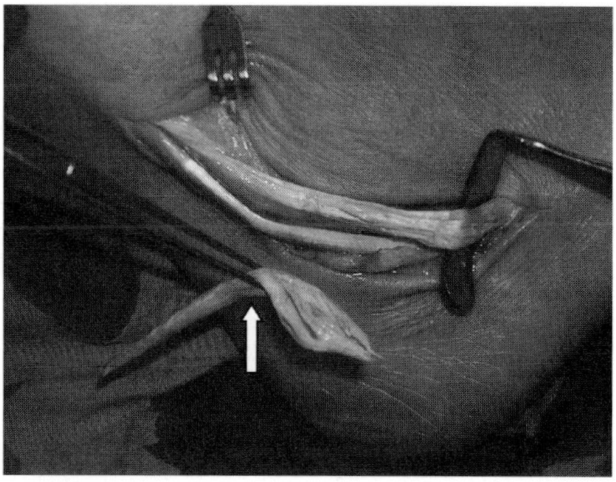

Fig. 8. A 3-cm longitudinal tear in the peroneus brevis has been treated by excision of the lateral 50% of the swollen tendon (*arrow*). The peroneus longus is normal. A synovectomy should be performed if necessary.

portion of the tendon when there is a tear may be a more reliable option than repair if adequate residual tendon tissue remains after debridement. Because no controlled studies compare suture and excision techniques, this question requires further research [27]. At the time of surgery, careful examination of the fibular groove is required to identify and deal with any osteophytes contributing to tendon abrasion. Appropriate repair of the superior peroneal retinaculum is also required in the presence of dislocation [16,22,27].

Degenerative ganglionic tears of the peroneus brevis at the level of the peroneal tubercle should include release and decompression of the thick fibrous tunnel at this level. If the peroneal tubercle is enlarged, consideration should be given to excising it to assist in decompression [32]. This is achieved by releasing the sheaths of both the brevis and longus to access the tubercle. Release with dissecting scissors rather than a scalpel reduces the risk of laceration of the underlying tendons at the level of the peroneal tubercle, as there is often associated stenosing tenosynovitis. Ganglionic tearing of the distal peroneus brevis does not usually require excision of tendon tissue, and is best dealt with by debridement and suture tubularization of the tendon.

Complete rupture of the peroneus brevis is ideally managed by primary repair. However, end-to-end repair is often not possible. In this case, the preferred surgical option depends on the integrity of the peroneus longus [16,22]. If the longus is intact, it can be sectioned at the cuboid tunnel and attached to the distal stump of the brevis as a tendon transfer. This option should be considered if there is a pes cavus with a plantarflexed first ray to reduce the moment of first metatarsal plantarflexion. A lateral-displacement calcaneal osteotomy may be necessary to neutralize a varus heel.

If the hindfoot is neutral, an alternative is to tenodese the peroneus longus to the distal stump of the brevis without dividing the longus. The decision to tenodese the peroneus longus to the brevis at the proximal limb depends on the integrity and excursion of the musculotendinous portion of the brevis. There is no advantage in tenodesing the peroneus longus to a scarred and fibrotic musculotendinous remnant proximally [27].

Acute peroneus longus tears may occur as a result of trauma or sport [10–12,17,31,34,35,47–53]. Lacerations of the peroneal tendons should be suspected even with small skin wounds. Any apparent weakness should be assessed to exclude or confirm damage. Acute surgical repair of a complete tendon laceration affords the patient the best chance of normal function. Longitudinal tears of the peroneus longus are less frequent than those of the brevis, but may coexist [22,27,31,47,54,55]. The surgical principles of repair outlined above apply.

Complete rupture of the peroneus longus most commonly occurs at the cuboid tunnel. If an os peroneum is present, rupture tends to occur immediately distal to this, but may involve fragmentation of the os peroneum, and this can be seen on plain radiographs. If complete rupture occurs in the presence of an os peroneum, the os peroneum may appear more proximal than usual on plain radiographs, a feature that assists in the diagnosis (Fig. 9) [35]. Complete peroneus longus rupture distally can be managed nonoperatively. However, if pain, swelling, and disability fail to improve, then debridement and transfer to the peroneus brevis is recommended [22]. Less common is the insertional tear of the peroneus longus presenting as pain deep in the midfoot after a sudden twisting injury or fall. This is seen best on MRI scanning, and should be managed nonoperatively.

There are several reports of acute ruptures of both peroneal tendons (Fig. 10) [22,53,56,57]. While end-to-end repair is preferred, this is not always possible, and the options then include a dynamic transfer of the flexor digitorum longus; an interposition graft, such as gracilis or semitendinosis; or a strip of iliotibial band to bridge the defect. Any of these options only succeed if there is adequate viability and excursion of the proximal musculature (Fig. 11). Wind and Rohrbacher [53] describe another approach involving reconstruction with the peroneal sheath and a peroneus tertius graft in a collegiate athlete. In this case, they employed the tenodesed proximal limbs of the peroneus longus and brevis that retained excursion.

Cross and Crichton [24] describe a rupture of the peroneus brevis in a classical ballet dancer found to have a congenitally absent peroneus longus muscle and tendon. Imaging showed an intact peroneus longus on the contralateral side. End-to-end repair was performed with a satisfactory return to dance.

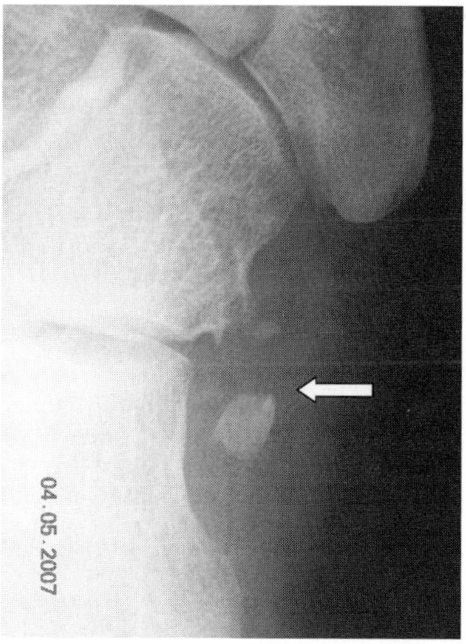

Fig. 9. Fragmentation of the os peroneum is evident, with proximal migration of the main fragment (*arrow*), indicating rupture of the peroneus longus. This bone is only present in 10% to 20% of the population.

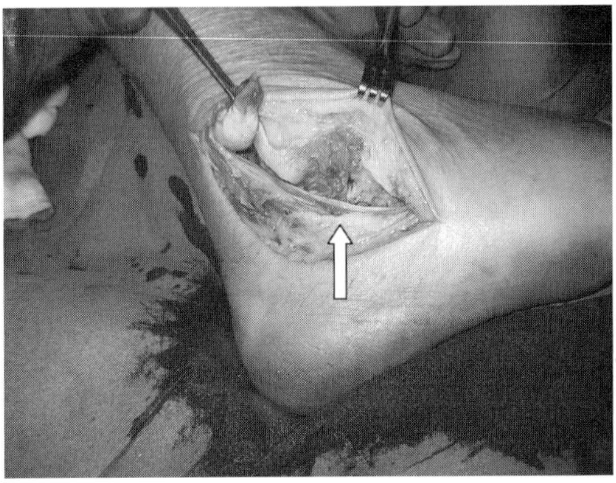

Fig. 10. Acute-on-chronic rupture of both peroneal tendons, with an empty synovitic peroneal sheath (*arrow*) and proximal retraction of the rounded tendon ends.

Results

Selmani and colleagues [27], in a recent review, stated that, to date, all studies outlining the surgical management of peroneal tendon tears are either retrospective reviews (level IV evidence) or case reviews (level V evidence), concluding that there is insufficient evidence to recommend for or against any specific treatment (grade I). A more recent study by Steel and DiOrio [58] found that only 46% of 30 patients treated surgically for peroneal tendon tears were able to successfully return to sports. At an average follow-up of 31 months, 58% had residual scar tenderness and 54% residual ankle swelling. Surgical treatment did allow 9 of 10 patients working outdoors to resume work.

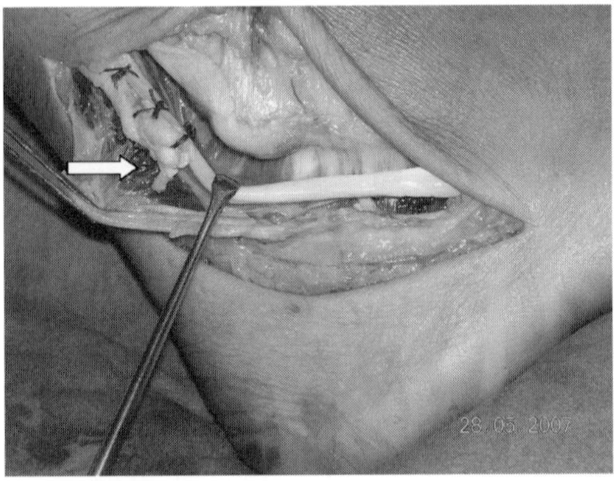

Fig. 11. Complete rupture of the peroneus longus and brevis, and a large defect. The flexor digitorum longus has been transferred from the medial side and attached to the distal stump of the brevis. As some excursion remained proximally, the peronei have been tenodesed to the transferred tendon (*arrow*).

It is clear that some peroneal tendon tears, if left untreated, progress to complete rupture with long-term progressive deformities. The decision to treat these lesions surgically, especially in the presence of acute tears, is based on sound biomechanical and surgical principles [16,17,22]. Controlled studies are required to determine preferred surgical methods and to confirm the need for correction of associated pathology, such as fibular groove deepening, excision of the peroneal tubercle, calcaneal osteotomy, and ankle stabilization. Studies of nonoperative treatment of dislocating peroneal tendons, however, are not justified, given the natural history of this abnormality.

Summary

Acute peroneal tendon tears lay at one end of a spectrum of peroneal tendon pathology, including peroneal tendonitis, peroneal tendon instability, stenosing peroneal tenosynovitis, and chronic peroneal tendon tears. Clinical awareness of the possibility of acute peroneal tendon pathology in association with other disorders of the foot and ankle is essential for making an accurate diagnosis and for formulating an appropriate management plan. Careful observation of swelling, tenderness, and weakness should alert the clinician to the possibility of peroneal tendon damage.

Because a tear represents a mechanical abnormality, surgical treatment is frequently required and should address not only the torn tendons, but also any underlying causative factor, such as dislocating peroneal tendons, stenosing peroneal tenosynovitis, an enlarged peroneal tubercle, a fragmented os peroneum, or an associated condition, such as ankle instability, ankle arthrosis, or pes cavus. Anatomical variants need to be considered as a potential cause of lateral ankle pain. Both high-quality ultrasonography and MRI scanning are helpful in the evaluation of these disorders. Most acute peroneus brevis tears are longitudinal, occur adjacent to the tip of the fibula, and require surgical treatment to correct the tear and associated pathology. Acute peroneus longus tears more commonly occur at the level of the cuboid tunnel and may initially be managed nonoperatively, but, if associated with stenosing tendonitis, may require debridement and tenodesis. Rarely, complete ruptures of both peronei occur and, if there is a significant defect, reconstructive procedures are required. Studies suggest that early diagnosis and surgical treatment of acute peroneal tendon tears can result in normal pain-free function, even in athletes. Controlled prospective studies of peroneal tendon tears will clarify preferred surgical treatment options.

References

[1] Sammarco GJ, Burstein AH, Frankel VH. Biomechanics of the ankle: a kinematic study. Orthop Clin North Am 1973;4(1):75–96.

[2] Davis WH, Sobel M, Deland J, et al. The superior peroneal retinaculum: an anatomic study. Foot Ankle Int 1994;15(5):271–5.
[3] Title CI, Jung HG, Parks BG, et al. The peroneal groove deepening procedure: a biomechanical study of pressure reduction. Foot Ankle Int 2005;26(6):442–8.
[4] Waitches GM, Rockett M, Brage M, et al. Ultrasonographic-surgical correlation of ankle tendon tears. J Ultrasound Med 1998;17(4):249–56.
[5] Sobel M, Levy ME, Bohne WH. Congenital variations of the peroneus quartus muscle: an anatomic study. Foot Ankle 1990;11(2):81–9.
[6] Cheung YY, Rosenberg ZS, Ramsinghani R, et al. Peroneus quartus muscle: MR imaging features. Radiology 1997;202(3):745–50.
[7] Saupe N, Mengiardi B, Pfirrmann CW, et al. Anatomic variants associated with peroneal tendon disorders: MR imaging findings in volunteers with asymptomatic ankles. Radiology 2007;242(2):509–17.
[8] Petersen W, Bobka T, Stein V, et al. Blood supply of the peroneal tendons: injection and immunohistochemical studies of cadaver tendons. Acta Orthop Scand 2000;71(2):168–74.
[9] Sobel M, Geppert MJ, Hannafin JA, et al. Microvascular anatomy of the peroneal tendons. Foot Ankle 1992;13(8):469–72.
[10] Bianchi S, Abdelwahab IF, Tegaldo G. Fracture and posterior dislocation of the os peroneum associated with rupture of the peroneus longus tendon. Can Assoc Radiol J 1991; 42(5):340–4.
[11] Peacock KC, Resnick EJ, Thoder JJ. Fracture of the os peroneum with rupture of the peroneus longus tendon. A case report and review of the literature. Clin Orthop Relat Res 1986; 202:223–6.
[12] Clarke HD, Kitaoka HB, Ehman RL. Peroneal tendon injuries. Foot Ankle Int 1998;19(5): 280–8.
[13] Brandes CB, Smith RW. Characterization of patients with primary peroneus longus tendinopathy: a review of twenty-two cases. Foot Ankle Int 2000;21(6):462–8.
[14] Bonnin M, Tavernier T, Bouysset M. Split lesions of the peroneus brevis tendon in chronic ankle laxity. Am J Sports Med 1997;25(5):699–703.
[15] Geppert MJ, Sobel M, Bohne WH. Lateral ankle instability as a cause of superior peroneal retinacular laxity: an anatomic and biomechanical study of cadaveric feet. Foot Ankle 1993; 14(6):330–4.
[16] Krause JO, Brodsky JW. Peroneus brevis tendon tears: pathophysiology, surgical reconstruction, and clinical results. Foot Ankle Int 1998;19(5):271–9.
[17] Sammarco GJ. Peroneal tendon injuries. Orthop Clin North Am 1994;25(1):135–45.
[18] Sobel M, Bohne WH, Levy ME. Longitudinal attrition of the peroneus brevis tendon in the fibular groove: an anatomic study. Foot Ankle 1990;11(3):124–8.
[19] Sobel M, DiCarlo EF, Bohne WH, et al. Longitudinal splitting of the peroneus brevis tendon: an anatomic and histologic study of cadaveric material. Foot Ankle 1991;12(3): 165–70.
[20] Sobel M, Geppert MJ, Olson EJ, et al. The dynamics of peroneus brevis tendon splits: a proposed mechanism, technique of diagnosis, and classification of injury. Foot Ankle 1992; 13(7):413–22.
[21] Sobel M, Geppert MJ, Warren RF. Chronic ankle instability as a cause of peroneal tendon injury. Clin Orthop Relat Res 1993;296:187–91.
[22] Redfern D, Myerson M. The management of concomitant tears of the peroneus longus and brevis tendons. Foot Ankle Int 2004;25(10):695–707.
[23] Bruce WD, Christofersen MR, Phillips DL. Stenosing tenosynovitis and impingement of the peroneal tendons associated with hypertrophy of the peroneal tubercle. Foot Ankle Int 1999; 20(7):464–7.
[24] Cross MJ, Crichton KJ, Gordon H, et al. Peroneus brevis rupture in the absence of the peroneus longus muscle and tendon in a classical ballet dancer: a case report. Am J Sports Med 1988;16(6):677–8.

[25] Geller J, Lin S, Cordas D, et al. Relationship of a low-lying muscle belly to tears of the peroneus brevis tendon. Am J Orthop 2003;32(11):541–4.
[26] Sammarco GJ. Longitudinal attrition of the peroneus brevis tendon in the fibular groove: an anatomic study. Foot Ankle 1991;11(4):249–51.
[27] Selmani E, Gjata V, Gjika E. Current concepts review: peroneal tendon disorders. Foot Ankle Int 2006;27(3):221–8.
[28] Eckert WR, Davis EA Jr. Acute rupture of the peroneal retinaculum. J Bone Joint Surg Am 1976;58(5):670–2.
[29] Lamm BM, Myers DT, Dombek M, et al. Magnetic resonance imaging and surgical correlation of peroneus brevis tears. J Foot Ankle Surg 2004;43(1):30–6.
[30] Major NM, Helms CA, Fritz RC, et al. The MR imaging appearance of longitudinal split tears of the peroneus brevis tendon. Foot Ankle Int 2000;21(6):514–9.
[31] Sammarco GJ. Peroneus longus tendon tears: acute and chronic. Foot Ankle Int 1995;16(5):245–53.
[32] Pierson JL, Inglis AE. Stenosing tenosynovitis of the peroneus longus tendon associated with hypertrophy of the peroneal tubercle and an os peroneum. A case report. J Bone Joint Surg Am 1992;74(3):440–2.
[33] Sobel M, Pavlov H, Geppert MJ, et al. Painful os peroneum syndrome: a spectrum of conditions responsible for plantar lateral foot pain. Foot Ankle Int 1994;15(3):112–24.
[34] Kilkelly FX, McHale KA. Acute rupture of the peroneal longus tendon in a runner: a case report and review of the literature. Foot Ankle Int 1994;15(10):567–9.
[35] Tehranzadeh J, Stoll DA, Gabriele OM. Case report 271. Posterior migration of the os peroneum of the left foot, indicating a tear of the peroneal tendon. Skeletal Radiol 1984;12(1):44–7.
[36] Grant TH, Kelikian AS, Jereb SE, et al. Ultrasound diagnosis of peroneal tendon tears. A surgical correlation. J Bone Joint Surg Am 2005;87(8):1788–94.
[37] Tjin ATER, Schweitzer ME, Karasick D. MR imaging of peroneal tendon disorders. AJR Am J Roentgenol 1997;168(1):135–40.
[38] Khoury NJ, el-Khoury GY, Saltzman CL, et al. Brevis tendon tears: MR imaging evaluation. Radiology 1996;200(3):833–41.
[39] Rademaker J, Rosenberg ZS, Delfaut EM, et al. Tear of the peroneus longus tendon: MR imaging features in nine patients. Radiology 2000;214(3):700–4.
[40] Rosenberg ZS, Beltran J, Cheung YY, et al. MR features of longitudinal tears of the peroneus brevis tendon. AJR Am J Roentgenol 1997;168(1):141–7.
[41] Rosenberg ZS, Cheung Y, Jahss MH. Computed tomography scan and magnetic resonance imaging of ankle tendons: an overview. Foot Ankle 1988;8(6):297–307.
[42] Bonnin M, Tavernier T, Bouysset M. Split lesions of the peroneus brevis tendon in chronic ankle laxity. Am J Sports Med 1997;25:699–703.
[43] Scholten PE, van Dijk CN. Tendoscopy of the peroneal tendons. Foot Ankle Clin 2006;11(2):415–20.
[44] Jerosch J, Aldawoudy A. Tendoscopic management of peroneal tendon disorders. Knee Surg Sports Traumatol Arthrosc 2007;15(6):806–10.
[45] Sammarco GJ, Idusuyi OB. Reconstruction of the lateral ankle ligaments using a split peroneus brevis tendon graft. Foot Ankle Int 1999;20(2):97–103.
[46] Sobel M, Warren RF, Brourman S. Lateral ankle instability associated with dislocation of the peroneal tendons treated by the Chrisman-Snook procedure. A case report and literature review. Am J Sports Med 1990;18(5):539–43.
[47] Bassett FH 3rd, Speer KP. Longitudinal rupture of the peroneal tendons. Am J Sports Med 1993;21(3):354–7.
[48] Evans JD. Subcutaneous rupture of the tendon of peroneus longus. Report of a case. J Bone Joint Surg Br 1966;48(3):507–9.
[49] Pelet S, Saglini M, Garofalo R, et al. Traumatic rupture of both peroneal longus and brevis tendons. Foot Ankle Int 2003;24(9):721–3.

[50] Ross G, Regan KJ, McDevitt ER, et al. Rupture of the peroneus longus tendon in a military athlete. Am J Orthop 1999;28(11):657–8.
[51] Thompson FM, Patterson AH. Rupture of the peroneus longus tendon. Report of three cases. J Bone Joint Surg Am 1989;71(2):293–5.
[52] Truong DT, Dussault RG, Kaplan PA. Fracture of the os peroneum and rupture of the peroneus longus tendon as a complication of diabetic neuropathy. Skeletal Radiol 1995;24(8): 626–8.
[53] Wind WM, Rohrbacher BJ. Peroneus longus and brevis rupture in a collegiate athlete. Foot Ankle Int 2001;22(2):140–3.
[54] Diaz GC, van Holsbeeck M, Jacobson JA. Longitudinal split of the peroneus longus and peroneus brevis tendons with disruption of the superior peroneal retinaculum. J Ultrasound Med 1998;17(8):525–9.
[55] Shoda E, Kurosaka M, Yoshiya S, et al. Longitudinal ruptures of the peroneal tendons. A report of a rugby player. Acta Orthop Scand 1991;62(5):491–2.
[56] Borton DC, Lucas P, Jomha NM, et al. Operative reconstruction after transverse rupture of the tendons of both peroneus longus and brevis. Surgical reconstruction by transfer of the flexor digitorum longus tendon. J Bone Joint Surg Br 1998;80(5):781–4.
[57] Abraham E, Stirnaman JE. Neglected rupture of the peroneal tendons causing recurrent sprains of the ankle. Case report. J Bone Joint Surg Am 1979;61(8):1247–8.
[58] Steel MW, DeOrio JK. Peroneal tendon tears: return to sports after operative treatment. Foot Ankle Int 2007;28(1):49–54.

ELSEVIER
SAUNDERS

Foot Ankle Clin N Am
12 (2007) 675–695

FOOT AND
ANKLE CLINICS

Surgical Treatment of Peroneal Tendon Tears

Natalie Squires, MD[a], Mark S. Myerson, MD[b], Cesar Gamba, MD[b,*]

[a] *InMotion Clinic, 1615 Delaware Street, Longview, WA 98632, USA*
[b] *The Institute for Foot and Ankle Reconstruction, Mercy Medical Center, 301 St Paul Place, Baltimore, MD 21202, USA*

The peroneal muscles function as dynamic stabilizers of the ankle and are important in proprioception independent of the status of the lateral ankle ligaments. Poor peroneal function can give patients a sense of instability, even in a mechanically stable ankle, and can cause persistent pain and swelling after an ankle injury. Although the true incidence of peroneal tendon tears is unknown, estimates range from 11% to 37% in cadaver dissections, and up to 30% in patients undergoing surgery for ankle instability [1–9]. Unlike what is seen with the Achilles and the posterior tibialis tendons, the peroneal tendons have good vascularity and are not prone to degeneration due to poor blood supply [6,8,10,11]. However, the peroneal tendons are like the Achilles and posterior tibialis tendons in that such diseases as diabetes mellitus, spondyloarthropathy, and rheumatoid arthritis can predispose to tendonitis. The etiology of peroneal tendon tears is primarily traumatic whether as an isolated process or associated with recurrent inversion sprains of the ankle. It is a mechanical problem with secondary degeneration demonstrating fibroblastic proliferation and disruption of the normal collagen architecture on histological evaluation [8]. The focus of this article is the diagnosis and treatment of peroneal tendon tears.

Mechanism of injury

An acute peroneal tendon dislocation or tearing occurs when the ankle sustains a sudden forced dorsiflexion accompanied by a concomitant reflexive contraction of the peroneal muscles [11–13]. Peroneal tendon tears result

* Corresponding author.
E-mail address: cenriquegamba@hotmail.com (C. Gamba).

doi:10.1016/j.fcl.2007.08.002

from inversion or recurrent inversion injuries to the ankle [3,9,11,13–18]. The mechanism of a peroneal tendon tear is the same as that of an ankle sprain. Anatomically, the superior peroneal retinaculum (SPR) acts as a secondary restraint to ankle inversion stress and its calcaneal branch runs parallel to the calcaneofibular ligament (CFL) [15,18]. An inversion injury may tear the CFL and injure the calcaneal branch of the SPR, causing attenuation and laxity of the retinaculum [3,7,9,15,17,18]. This laxity leads to tendon subluxation with mechanical abrasion of the peroneus brevis tendon against the posterior lip of the fibula or against the peroneus longus.

The association between inversion stress, lateral ankle ligament sprain, and peroneal tendinopathy accounts for the multiple reports of peroneal tendinopathy in patients with mechanical ankle instability [3,6,7,14,17,19]. When patients with peroneal tears are evaluated, 43% complain of instability and 66% have radiographic evidence of increased tilt on varus stress [5]. Peroneal tendon injury is in the differential diagnosis of lateral ankle sprains in patients complaining of chronic lateral ankle pain after an inversion injury.

Peroneal brevis tears

Peroneal brevis tears most commonly occur in the region of the peroneal sulcus in the posterior and distal region of the fibula [5–7,18,20–22]. Situated between the peroneus longus and the posterolateral fibula, the brevis is under significant stress and longitudinal tearing of the peroneal brevis can result from mechanical abrasion against the peroneus longus or against the posterolateral lip of the fibula as the SPR becomes incompetent [1,7,8,10,15,16,18].

A longitudinal tear is the most commonly seen tear in the peroneus brevis (Fig. 1), but occasionally a "bucket handle" tear (Fig. 2) of the peroneus

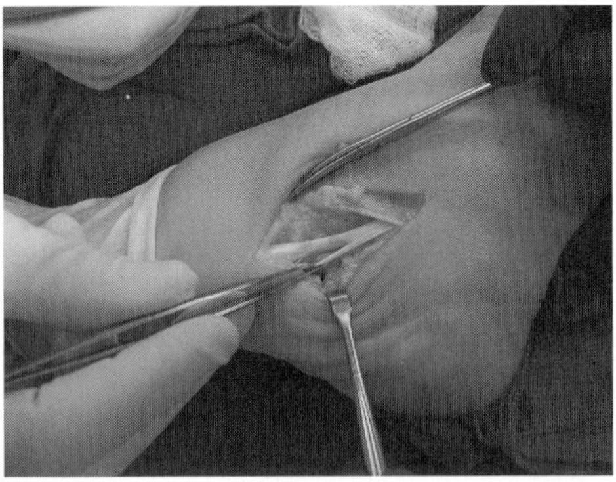

Fig. 1. Longitudinal split in the peroneal brevis tendon.

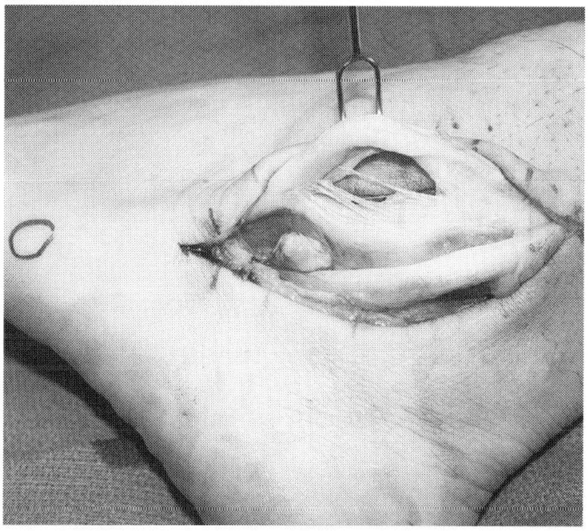

Fig. 2. "Bucket handle" tear of peroneal brevis tendon.

brevis tendon may occur whereby the tendon splits and the peroneus longus acts like a wedge, lying between the split portions of the peroneus brevis [13].

Tears may also occur from a volume effect of increased pressure within the peroneal tunnel in the presence of a peroneus quartus or a low-lying peroneal brevis muscle belly [13]. The additional tissue bulk increases compression on the tendons because of overcrowding, and the relative risk of a peroneal brevis tear doubles in the presence of an anomalous peroneus quartus [7]. The peroneus brevis can also be injured at its insertion during an inversion foot injury that results in a fracture of the base of the fifth metatarsal.

Peroneal longus tears

Tears of the peroneus longus are much less frequent than those of the brevis tendon. Like tears of the peroneus brevis, tears of the peroneus longus tendon occur in areas of high stress. The peroneus longus tendon changes direction three times before it inserts into the medial cuneiform. The most acute, or angular, change occurs at the plantar aspect of the cuboid. Brandes [23] categorized three zones along the longus tendon: Zone A extends from the tip of the malleolus to the peroneal tubercle, zone B from the lateral trochlear process to the inferior retinaculum, and zone C from the inferior retinaculum to the cuboid notch. Zone C is a high-stress area, particularly at the cuboid notch, and is the location of the majority of longus tears [23,24]. In a patient who presents with acute pain on the inferior and lateral aspect of the foot, the presence of an os peroneum (present in 20% of patients) should call attention to a possible peroneus longus injury, though the absence of an os peroneum does not preclude an injury to the longus tendon [24]. A multipartite os peroneum occurs in 25% patients and, as with other sesamoids, may make the diagnosis of a fracture difficult. Although peroneus brevis tears are far more common, more deformity is seen with longus tears because of its size and function as a pronator of the foot. Chronic rupture of the peroneus longus, with or without a brevis tear, can lead to a cavovarus deformity [5,23,25].

Associated pathology

Ankle instability

The association between ankle instability and peroneal tendinopathy is well known.

According to DiGiovanni and colleagues [3] peroneal synovitis is seen in 77%, retinacular attenuation in 54%, and longitudinal brevis tears in 25% of patients with chronic lateral ankle instability. The presence of mechanical instability to varus stress indicates a rupture of the anterior talofibular ligament, CFL, or both. A mechanically unstable ankle is prone to recurrent inversion sprains, which also potentially injures the peroneal tendons. As dynamic stabilizers of the ankle, the peroneals can increase lateral ankle stability. However, if they are injured, they cannot effectively "pick up the slack" of the ruptured ankle ligaments.

When examining a patient with frank mechanical instability, one tends to focus on the torn lateral ankle ligaments and the peroneal tendons can easily be overlooked as a source of persistent pain. A patient with an unstable ankle presents with symptoms as such (ie, instability) and not pain. If pain is present, then one has to start sorting out where and why. The most common cause of pain is a torn peroneal tendon. For this reason, reconstruction of the ankle ligaments alone, without addressing the peroneal tendons, will not be successful. Similarly, addressing the tendons alone without correcting the mechanical instability only increases the stresses placed on the peroneal tendons, thereby increasing the likelihood of failure. Forty-three percent of patients with peroneal tendinopathy complain of instability in the affected ankle. Of these patients, 66% demonstrate clinical instability on drawer and tilt testing, and radiographic instability on varus stress [5].

Hindfoot varus

In neurologically compromised patients, chronic peroneal weakness results in cavovarus deformity as a result of posterior tibialis overpull [25]. This process also occurs in neurologically normal patients in the presence of a varus hindfoot deformity, which is commonly associated with an increased incidence of ankle instability and peroneal tears. Hindfoot varus places increased stress on the stabilizing structures in the lateral ankle, and patients are at an increased risk of recurrent inversion sprains. Failure to recognize and to correct the hindfoot alignment results in recurrent ankle inversion sprains.

The presence of hindfoot varus caused by chronic ruptures of the peroneal tendons has been described [16]. Clearly, the presence of hindfoot varus is integral to the outcome of treatment of a rupture of the peroneal tendon, whether the cause or the effect of the deformity.

Hypertrophied peroneal tubercle

The peroneal tendons pass anterior to the tubercle as they course along the lateral calcaneus. Hypertrophy of the tubercle causes stenosis and mechanical irritation of the tendons, leading to tendonitis, tearing, and frequently rupture. The reason why the peroneal tubercle is seen more commonly in patients with a cavus foot deformity is a topic of speculation. The peroneal tubercle must be addressed when performing repair or release of the peroneal tendons. There is commonly a stenosis of one or both of the tendons as they pass in front of or behind the tubercle, and an hourglass deformity of the tendon is noted. At times, simple release of the tendon sheath with removal of the hypertrophied peroneal tubercle is all that is needed to alleviate symptoms. The sheath of both tendons is opened, an ostectomy of the tubercle is performed, and the underlying cancellous bone smoothed with bone wax to prevent further irritation.

Diagnosis

Clinically, the patient presents with a history of an "ankle sprain" that never fully resolves. Frequently patients complain of persistent posterolateral pain and a sense of instability. Posterolateral pain and swelling are the most reliable diagnostic signs [5,10,13,26].

Usually the diagnosis of peroneal tendon injury is obvious, with swelling laterally, pain to palpation along the course of the tendons, and crepitation to resisted eversion. Passive inversion or adduction may elicit pain by placing stress on tendons. The presence of strong and painless resisted eversion does not rule out the diagnosis of a peroneal tendon tear because the remaining tendon (if normal) can completely compensate for the lack of function of the other. Pain is frequently present, however, with active eversion, as well as with extreme passive dorsiflexion. Pain can be reproduced with the patient standing with the involved foot posteriorly, and then leaning forward as if to do a "runner's stretch." Compression of the SPR during active or resisted eversion may also reproduce peroneal pain. Check for balance and stability on single- and double-heel rise. All patients should perform a test of proprioception, which is an attempt to stand on one foot with the eyes closed. Tilt and anterior drawer testing should be performed to diagnose any mechanical ankle instability. Hindfoot alignment should be evaluated for the presence of a varus deformity, and a routine test of the mobility of the medial column of the foot performed with the Coleman block test if any hindfoot varus is noted.

Several findings are key to the diagnosis:

Swelling posterolaterally along the course of the tendons
Pain on palpation along the course of the tendon
Pain exacerbated by compression of the SPR as the patient actively everts the ankle [9]
Crepitation or squeaking of the tendons [9]
Pain with extreme active dorsiflexion, which compresses the SPR against the tendons [9]
Difficulty maintaining stability on single-stance heel rise [27]
Retromalleolar pain with anterior drawer testing [1]

Objective studies

Standing radiographs should include three views of the ankle and three views of the foot. Alignment can be assessed on the lateral view of the foot using Meary's line and assessing the height of the fifth metatarsal relative to the first metatarsal. Close evaluation of the ankle may diagnose the presence of a rim fracture of the distal fibula [12]. A base of the fifth metatarsal fracture or nonunion should prompt a careful evaluation for pain at the insertion of the brevis tendon. Spurs laterally at the calcaneus in patients with a history of calcaneus fracture may be a cause of tendon pain distal to the tip of the fibula. The os peroneum is normally located at the cuboid notch. Fracture or migration of the os peroneum should alert the surgeon to the possibility of a peroneus longus tendon tear or rupture (Fig. 3). Varus stress views of the ankle should reveal any mechanical instability due to rupture of the lateral ankle ligaments.

While MRI is not a useful examination for diagnosis of the extent of rupture, it certainly is a sensitive study for evaluation of the soft tissues around the ankle. Fluid around the peroneal tendon with normal signal within the tendon is indicative of tendonitis. Signal change within the substance of the tendon, enlargement of the tendon, or loss of tendon continuity indicates tendinopathy. Despite this, MRI is somewhat unreliable as a diagnostic tool for the diagnosis of peroneal tendon tears because it has been associated with a significant number of both false-positive and false-negative readings [3,5,10,23,26]. The authors have repeatedly found that the MRI either under- or overestimates the extent of peroneal tendon pathology that is subsequently identified intraoperatively. In one study, however, Bonnin and colleagues [1] found that in patients whose symptoms consisted primarily of pain without instability, MRI was a helpful tool. Particularly useful were the proton density images of the tendons in the transverse plane [1]. Additional findings on MRI include a hypertrophied peroneal tubercle, which is readily seen on T2-weighted images. It is associated with bony edema (Fig. 4). Because of the unreliability of MRI studies, and the ease of diagnosis with correct physical examination, the diagnosis of a peroneal tendon tear is

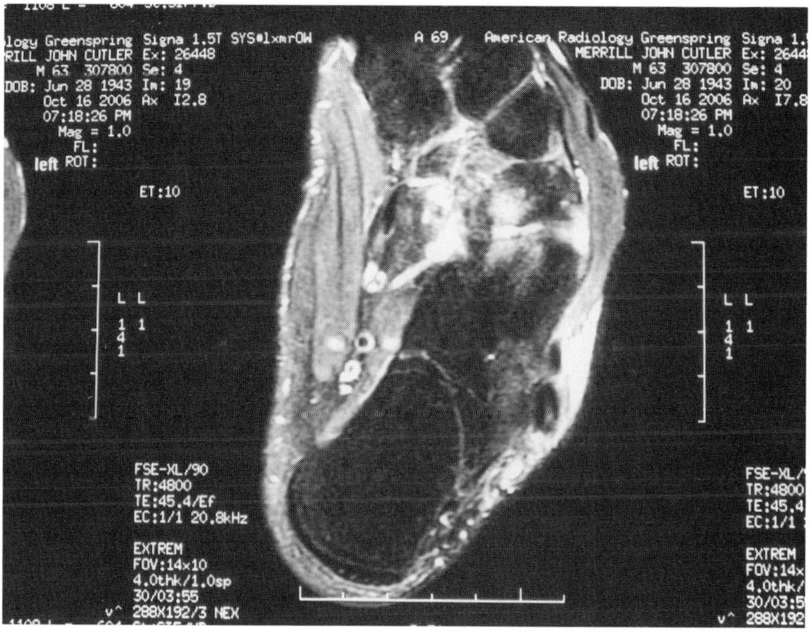

Fig. 3. Bony edema and tendon signal change at the peroneal tubercle.

largely clinical, and MRI should only be used to establish that some "pathology" of the tendon or tendons may be present.

Conservative treatment

Conservative treatment consists of anti-inflammatory medications, lateral heel wedge, bracing, and physical therapy. Although these modalities are useful for the treatment of tendonitis, they are not successful for the treatment of an established tear and the failure rate is very high. Furthermore, once torn, the likelihood of the rupture worsening is present and, as the pathologic process increases, the treatment options become more complicated. Thus, the management of an acute or chronic tear of the peroneal tendon is largely surgical and should be considered in patients who have either acute or chronic pain, instability, and decreased function [5,7,23,27].

Operative treatment

Isolated peroneus brevis tear

Given that the diagnosis of peroneal tears is largely clinical, often the extent of the injury is not known before surgical exploration. The type of

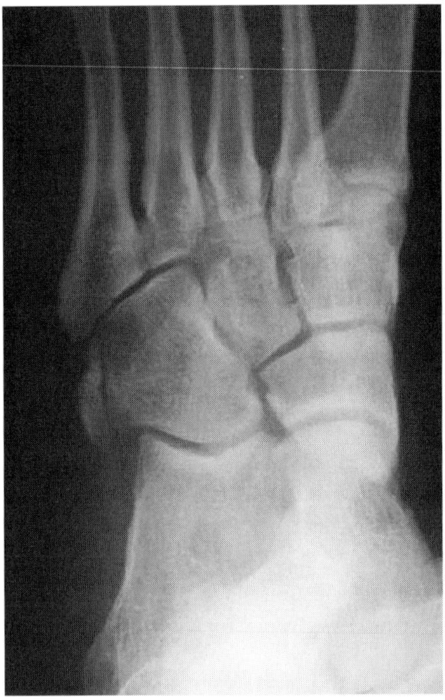

Fig. 4. Os peroneum.

repair undertaken is therefore based on the surgical findings. The retinaculum is inspected to assess for rupture or laxity, and the tendons are inspected for continuity and for tears that are frequently noted on the posterior surface of the tendon. If the tendon appears grossly normal, flip the tendon to examine the posterior surface as well. The presence of a low-lying brevis muscle belly or a peroneus quartus is noted and excised to decompress the tunnel [9,10].

A slightly curved 8- to10-cm incision is made posterior to the lateral malleolus over the course of the peroneal tendons. The sural nerve must be identified and retracted, particularly if one is treating a more distal rupture because the nerve crosses the tendons more distally. The retinaculum is assessed for redundancy or elevation off of the lateral surface of the fibula. The ankle is taken through a range of motion to assess for subluxation. When the retinaculum is opened longitudinally, leave a 4-mm cuff of tissue anteriorly so that repair can be performed without constriction of the tendons. If present, inflamed synovial tissue, a good indicator of a rupture, should be removed. Once the area of the tear is identified, fibrous and loose fragmented tissue is resected. Small longitudinal tears that result in splaying with minimal degeneration or fraying are repaired with tubularization of the tendon using a running 4–0 absorbable suture (Fig. 5). If the viable portion of the tendon comprises greater than 50% of the tendon diameter (grade 1),

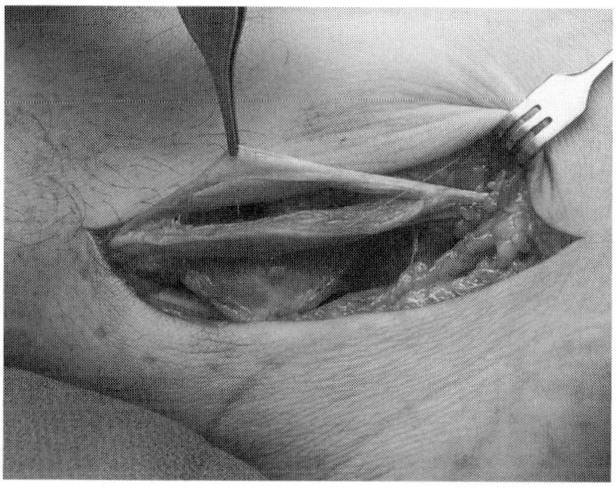

Fig. 5. Longitudinal split of the peroneus brevis.

then the degenerated portion should be completely excised and the viable tendon repaired longitudinally with a running 4–0 absorbable suture. Before excising the torn portion of the tendon, make sure that the ankle is stable. If the ankle is unstable, a nonanatomic procedure using the torn anterior portion of the peroneal tendon can be performed instead of resection. Tubularizing the tendon reestablishes a smooth tendon [6,19,20,28,29] (Fig. 6). If the viable portion of the tendon is less than 50% of the cross-sectional area (grade 2), then the degenerated portion is debrided and a proximal and distal tenodesis of the brevis tendon to the longus tendon can be performed with 2-0 absorbable suture [6,15,20,28]. An absorbable suture is used to avoid persistent irritation within the tendon sheath. To avoid fibula impingement, the proximal tenodesis is placed at least 3 to 4 cm above the tip of the lateral malleolus, and the distal tenodesis is placed at least 5 to 6 cm below the tip of the lateral malleolus. One has to be careful with this tenodesis because the scarring created particularly distally may lead

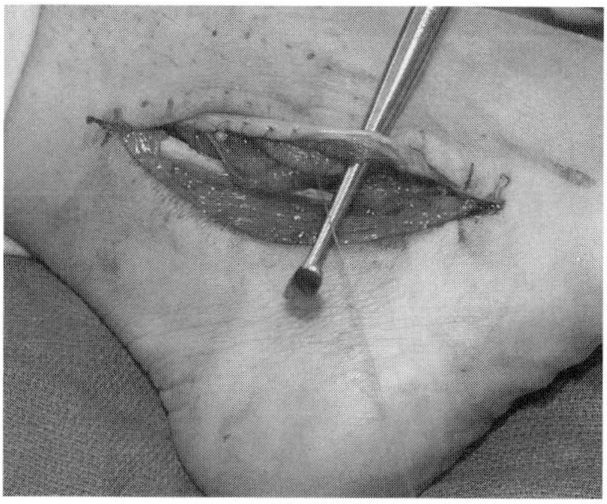

Fig. 6. Tubularization of the tendon after debridement.

to further tendon tearing and functional loss. There is no realistic alternative, however, to this tenodesis, but the authors' recommendation is to limit this to a suture proximal and not distal to the fibula.

Chronic attritional rupture of the insertion of the peroneus brevis tendon may require debridement of the tendon insertion and repair of the tendon using suture anchors. An anchor may be unnecessary if there is sufficient adjacent fibrous tissue for reattachment of the tendon. Sometimes there is a significant chronic degenerative rupture of the insertion of the brevis tendon, and if the gap precludes repair or reattachment, then it advisable to perform a tenodesis of the brevis to the longus tendon. This can be done either by cutting the longus and transferring it into the base of the fifth metatarsal or performing a side-to-side tenodesis, which as noted may cause additional scarring (Fig. 7).

The superior peroneal retinaculum is repaired either by direct suture or, if totally incompetent, by advancing the posterior flap and securing it through a series of drill holes in the posterolateral margin of the fibula. The anterior flap of the SPR is then brought posteriorly and sutured to the posterior flap to reinforce it. The foot is immobilized in a removable boot for 6 weeks and a removable stirrup splint is used for another 4 weeks. Active range of motion is starting at 3 weeks. At 4 weeks, full bearing of weight begins, depending on the extent of the tear and the need for additional tenodesis.

Isolated peroneus longus tear

If a simple longitudinal tear is present, a repair is performed after debridement of the lesion using a 4-0 absorbable suture as described above. However, if the tear is partial or complete but under or adjacent to the cuboid, a more difficult decision must be made. Ideally, if an os peroneum is present and fractured, part of this or all the bone is excised and a repair is made using an end-to-end correction or performing a tubularization of the remaining tendon (Figs. 8 and 9). This is easier said than done, however,

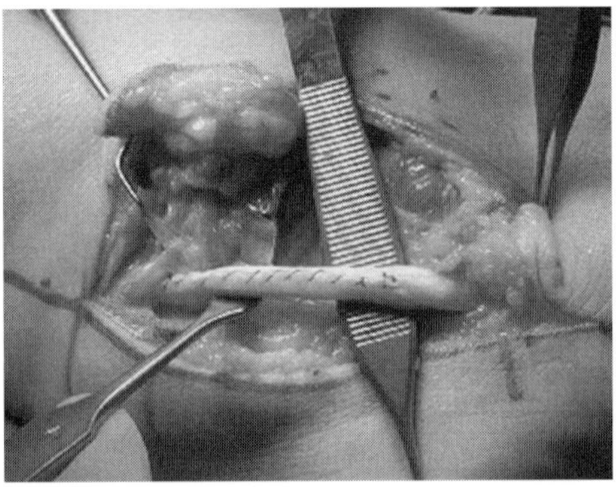

Fig. 7. Tubularization of the tendon.

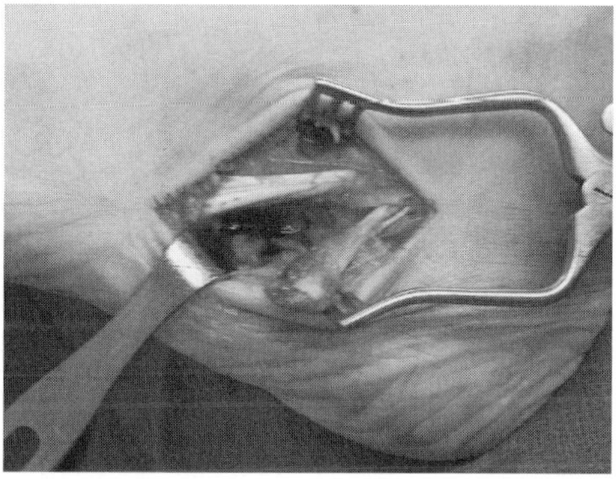

Fig. 8. Rupture of peroneus longus at the os peroneum.

because the dissection under the cuboid is difficult. The incision has to be extended further distally, and the abductor muscle retracted inferiorly. If the tendon ends can be approximated or there remains tendon in continuity, then this repair is ideal. Once, however, the rupture is complete there is a tendency for proximal retraction, which may preclude any end-to-end repair. Usually the rupture is located underneath the cuboid, but it may be more proximal, as seen in the presence of a hypertrophied peroneal tubercle. Once the stump is identified, the degenerated area is debrided, leaving as much length as possible, and tendon excursion is assessed. Whenever possible, a direct repair of the tendon is recommended, using a 4-0 fiber wire suture.

If there is excursion, but not enough tendon length for an end-to-end repair, then the longus tendon can be attached to the lateral border of the cuboid using a biointerference screw (Fig. 10). If there is tendon excursion, but not enough length to reach the cuboid, then a tenodesis is the ideal treatment and this is performed with a side-to-side technique to the peroneus

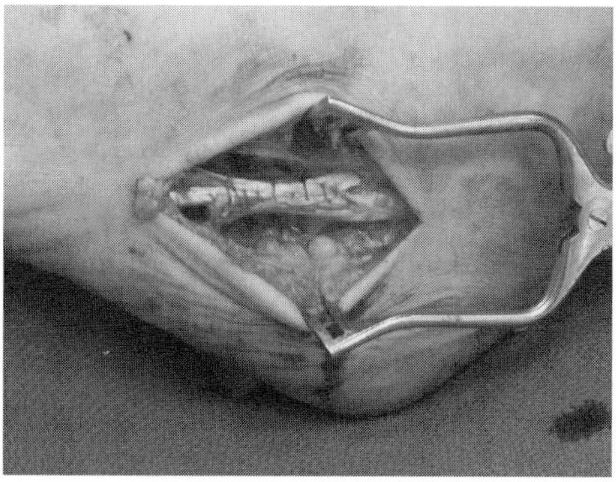

Fig. 9. Tenodesis of peroneus longus to the peroneus brevis.

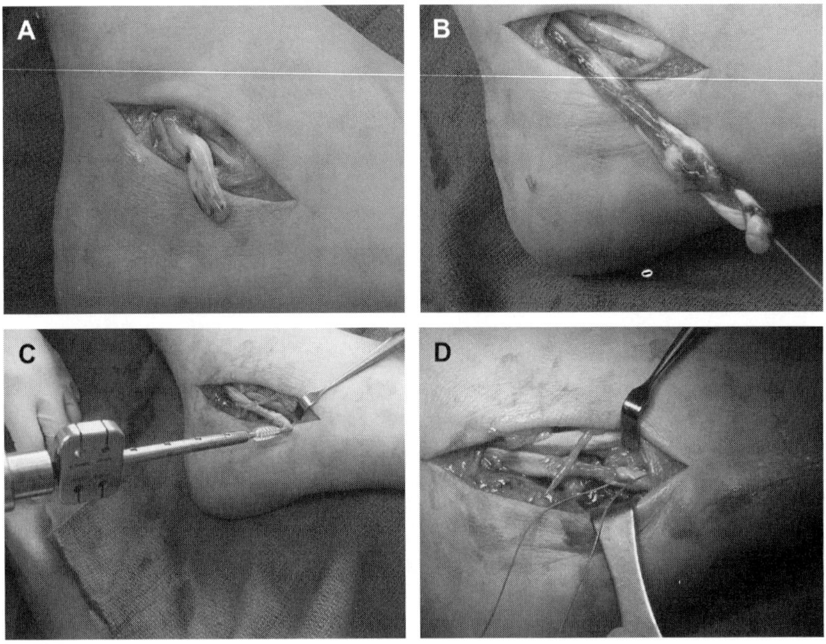

Fig. 10. A 32-year-old professional baseball player. (*A*) Isolated acute peroneus longus tear. (*B*) Preparation of tendon. (*C*) Preparation of the tunnel in the cuboid bone for bio-interference screw. (*D*) Repaired peroneus longus tendon.

brevis. If there is no excursion of the proximal stump whatsoever, then a tenodesis could lock up a functional peroneus brevis tendon and should not be performed. The tenodesis of the longus to the brevis is performed with a running absorbable 4-0 fiber wire suture used in a side-to-side fashion over a length of 2 to 3 cm to gain as much control of the tendon as possible. Avoid any bulk on the distal portion of the incision.

Tears of both the peroneus longus and brevis

The treatment of combined tears of the peroneus longus and brevis has been previously described by Redfern and Myerson [5] and is based on a validated protocol (Fig. 11).

As with isolated tears of the peroneus brevis and longus, the type of rupture and the amount of tendon degeneration must be assessed intraoperatively.

If both tendons are grossly intact (type I), they are repaired in a standard manner by excising the longitudinal tear and tubularizing the remaining tendon with a running 4-0 suture. If one tendon is completely torn and irreparable, but the other tendon is considered functional (type II), then a tenodesis is done proximally using musculotendinous tissue and any

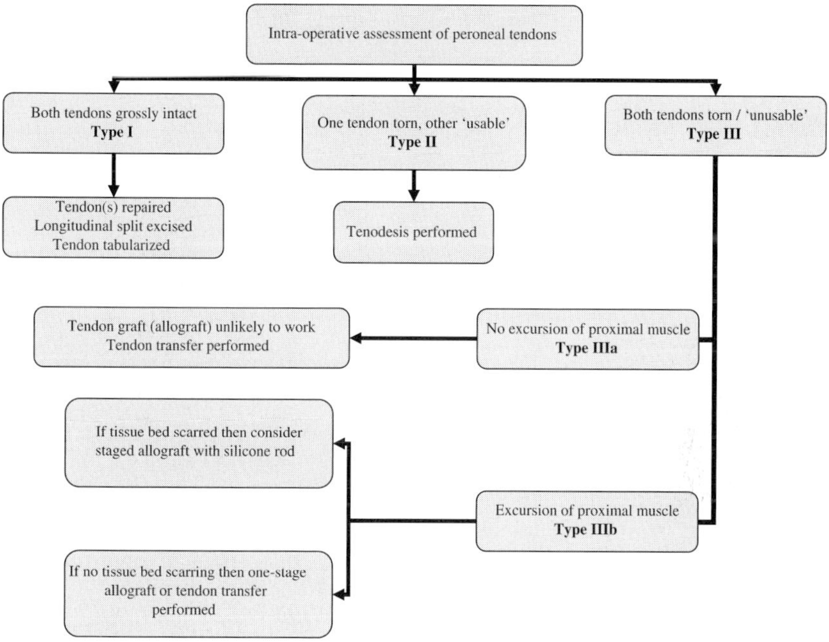

Fig. 11. Validated protocol on the treatment of combined tears of the peroneus longus and brevis. (*From* Redfern D, Myerson M. The management of concomitant tears of the peroneus longus and brevis tendons. Foot Ankle Int 2004;25:695–707; with permission)

healthy tendon distal to the muscle (Figs. 12 and 13). The decision to include a tenodesis is based on the state of the muscle. As with isolated tears, a tenodesis is not recommended if muscle excursion of either tendon is absent secondary to scarring and presumed muscle fibrosis.

If the both tendons are nonfunctional (type III), then a tendon graft or tendon transfer of the flexor digitorum longus (FDL) to the peroneus brevis is recommended. This decision is based on the amount of excursion of the

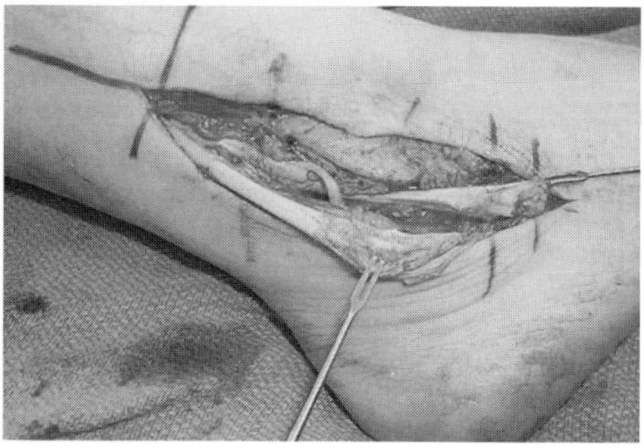

Fig. 12. One tendon is not "usable."

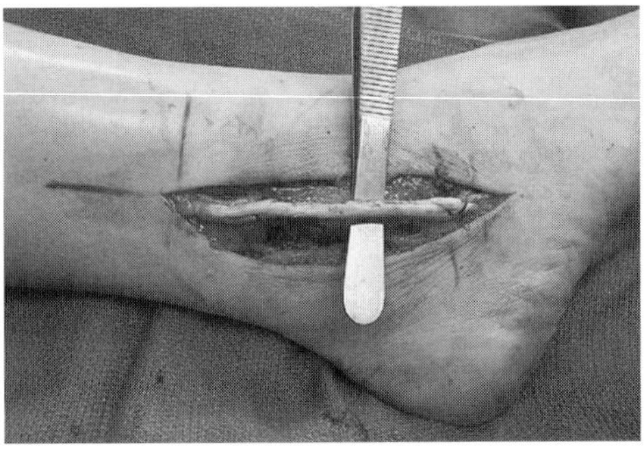

Fig. 13. Tenodesis of peroneus brevis to peroneus longus.

muscle proximally (Figs. 14 and 15). If no excursion of the proximal muscle is evident (type IIIa), then an FDL transfer is the procedure of choice. If there is tendon excursion (type IIIb), then an allograft tendon reconstruction is the procedure of choice.

Either procedure can be performed in one or two stages, depending on the state of the tendon bed. After excision of the degenerated tendon, the tendon bed is assessed for scarring. If minimal or no scarring is present, then the procedure of choice can be performed in the same setting. If scarring is present, then the surgery must be staged. The first stage reestablishes a synovialized cavity with the use of a silicone rod (2,3).

Silicone rod technique

With the silicone rod technique, a longitudinal incision is made 5 cm proximal and 6 cm distal to the tip of the fibula over the course of the peroneal tendons. The excursion and function of the tendons are checked. In patients with severe scar and retraction, sometimes it is difficult to

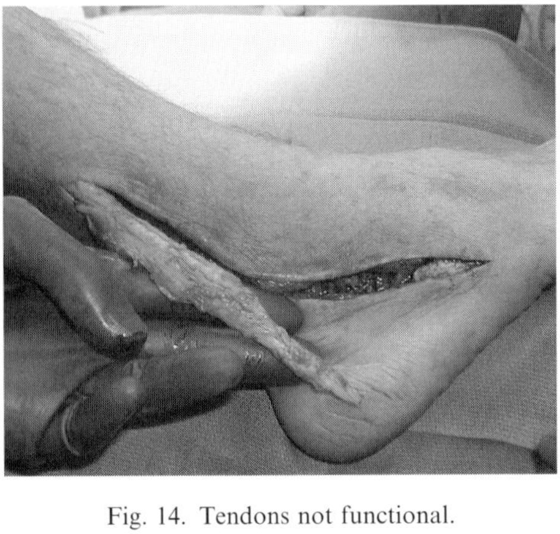

Fig. 14. Tendons not functional.

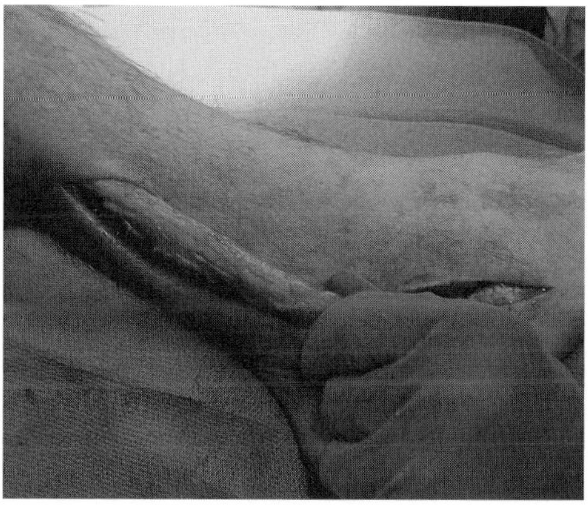

Fig. 15. No tendon excursion.

distinguish between the peroneus brevis and longus. If some excursion of the muscle tendinous unit is still present, then an allograft tendon reconstruction is planned. If, because of muscle fibrosis, there is no excursion of the tendon, then an FDL transfer is planned. The degenerated tendon is excised leaving a small stump proximally and distally. After excision of the scarred tendons, the tendon bed is assessed for scarring. If scarring is present, a silicone rod is inserted and attached distally to the remaining stump of the peroneus brevis tendon (Figs. 16 and 17). The proximal end is left free to allow for motion of the rod [30]. The incision is closed and early motion is allowed. The procedure of choice is performed 6 weeks later once there is a synovialized cavity.

Hamstring allograft reconstruction

As a single-stage procedure, the allograft reconstruction is relatively straightforward. After excision of the degenerated tendon, a hamstring allograft is attached to the proximal muscle and tendon using #2 fiber wire suture. The foot is held in maximal eversion during insertion of the tendon distally. If there is a substantial brevis stump, then the allograft is sutured

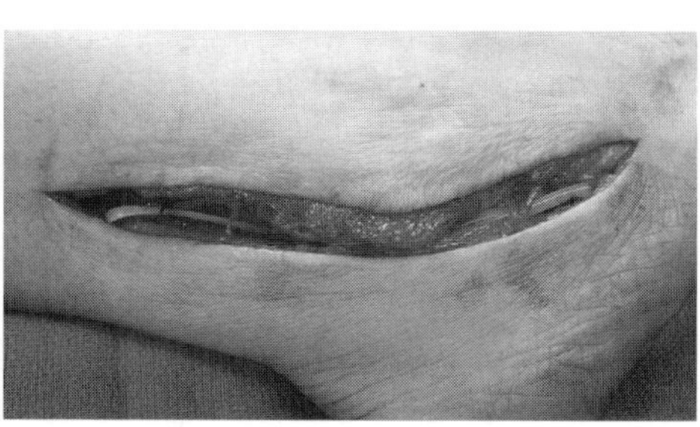

Fig. 16. Silicone rod placement.

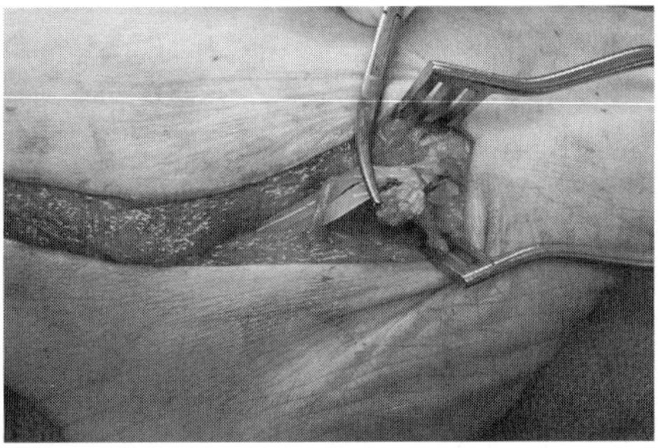

Fig. 17. Attachment of the rod distally to the stump of the peroneus brevis.

into the distal tendon. However, loss of viable tendon may necessitate insertion into the base of the fifth metatarsal with suture anchors.

The incision for a staged hamstring allograft reconstruction is different than that for a primary reconstruction. Two incisions are made; the proximal incision exposes only the rod–tendon junction, and the distal incision exposes only the attachment site distally. The proximal incision is slightly longer than the distal incision. This technique avoids opening the entire wound and preserves the synovialized cavity created over the silicone rod. Once the proximal silicone stump is exposed, the hamstring allograft is attached to the myotendinous junction, and the distal end is attached to the free end of the silicone rod. The distal incision is made and, as the rod is removed through the distal wound, it draws the distal tendon into the synovialized cavity and down to the fifth metatarsal base (Fig. 18) [30]. The tendon is attached then distally to the base of the fifth metatarsal with a suture anchor (Fig. 19), or to the distal brevis stump. It is important to apply adequate tension to the allograft.

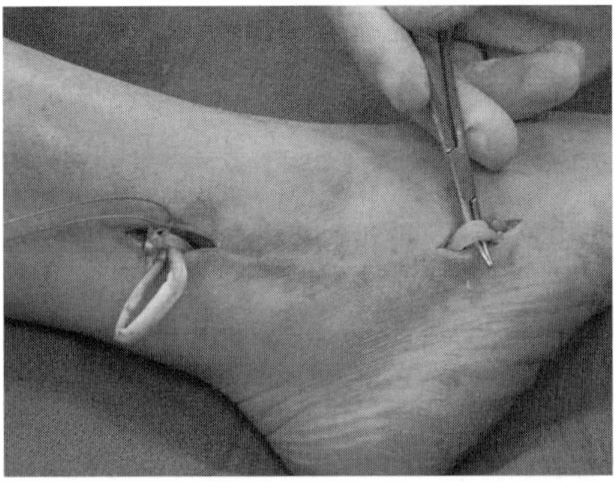

Fig. 18. Staged allograft reconstruction of the peroneal tendons. Note the small proximal and distal incisions.

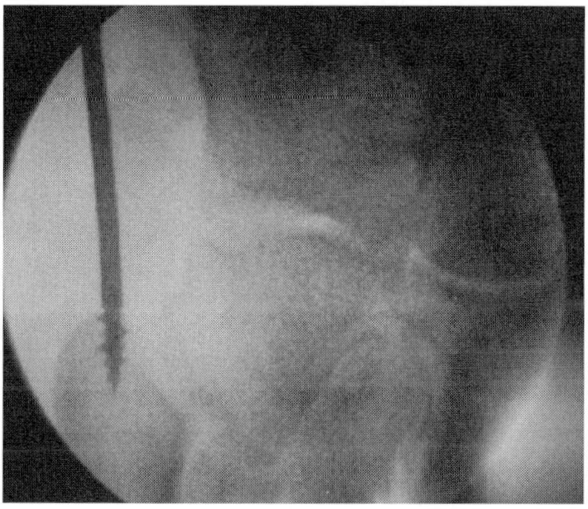

Fig. 19. Attachment of the tendon graft to the base of the fifth metatarsal.

Flexor digitorum longus transfer to the peroneus brevis

In a single-stage procedure, the FDL tendon is harvested after excision of the degenerated peroneal tendon. On the medial side, a double approach is used to expose the FDL. A small 1- or 2-cm incision is made just below the medial portion of the abductor hallucis muscle on the plantar medial aspect of the midfoot (Fig. 20). The FDL is identified at the master knot of Henry and followed distally. The tendon is transected as distally as possible to maintain length. A tenodesis of the FDL to the flexor hallucis longus before transection of the FDL is not necessary. The tendon is tagged with a Kessler-type suture. A second smaller incision is made proximal and posterior to the medial malleolus. The sheath over the FDL is opened and the tendon is pulled proximally (Fig. 21). It is then rerouted from medial across the deep

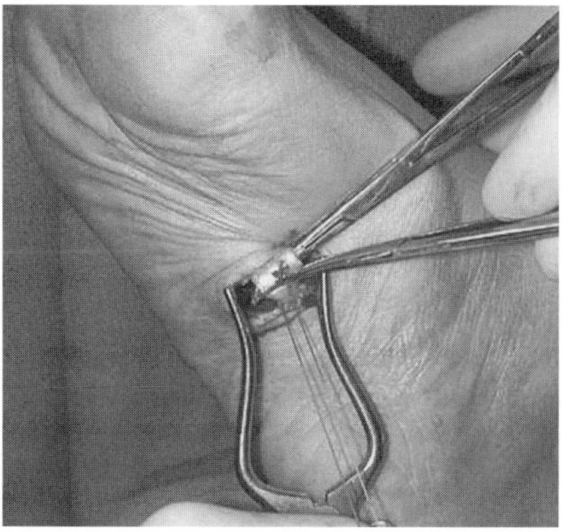

Fig. 20. Medial plantar incision for harvest of the FDL tendon.

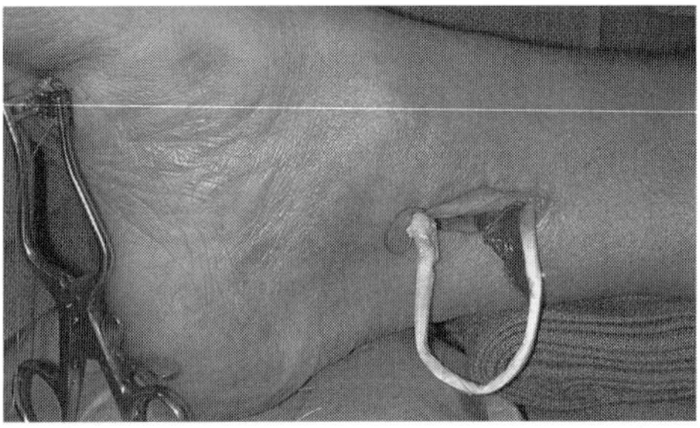

Fig. 21. The FDL is pulled proximally.

compartment, posterior to the neurovascular bundle and anterior to the Achilles tendon, to the lateral fibula and into the incision (Figs. 22 and 23) [30]. It is then routed along the peroneal brevis tendon bed and attached to the base of the fifth metatarsal with the foot in maximal eversion.

As part of the staged procedure, a small incision is made in the proximal and distal aspects of the lateral wound, identical to that in the staged allograft procedure. After retrieval of the tendon to the posterior medial malleolus, the tendon is routed laterally, posterior to the neurovascular bundle and anterior to the Achilles tendon. The tendon is introduced into the proximal lateral incision and tied to the silicone rod, which is then removed through the distal incision, thereby transferring the FDL tendon into the synovialized cavity (Fig. 24). The rod is then removed from its attachment to the FDL, and the tendon is attached to the base of the fifth metatarsal via suture anchors while the foot is held in maximal eversion.

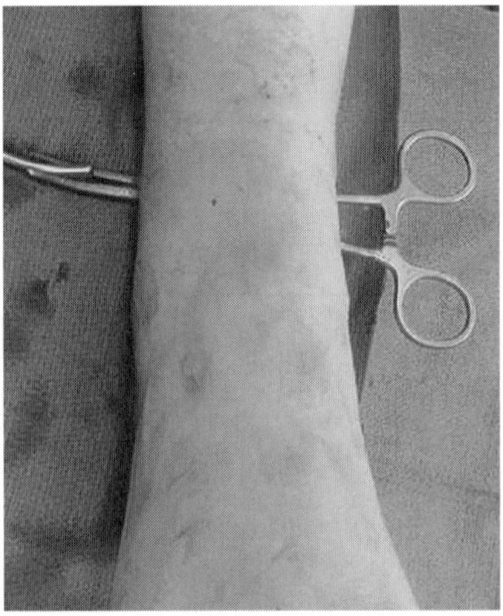

Fig. 22. Lateral transfer of the tendon.

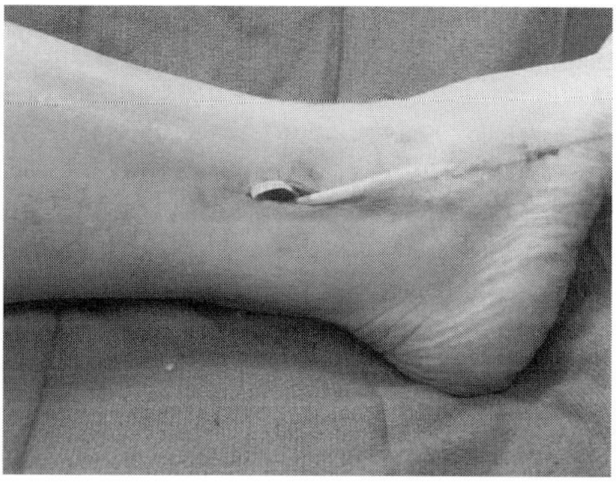

Fig. 23. The FDL is pulled into the proximal lateral wound.

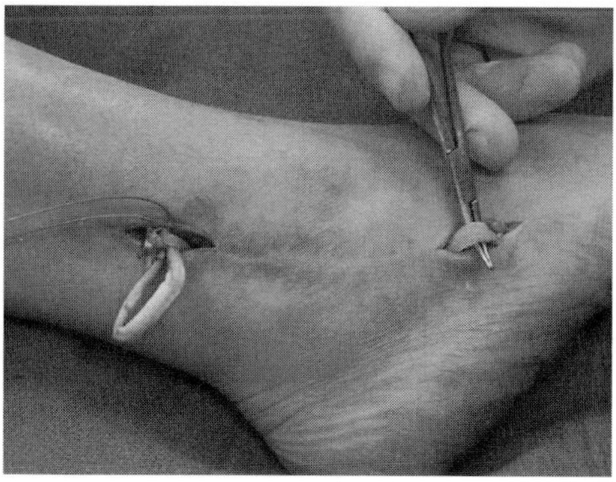

Fig. 24. The tendon is transferred into the synovialized cavity by removing the silicone rod through the distal wound

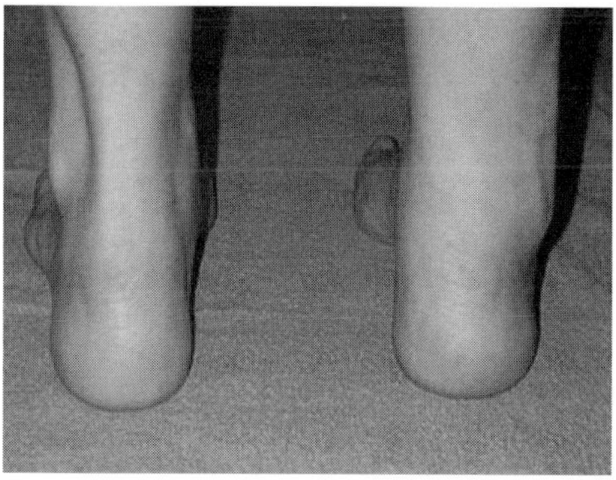

Fig. 25. Right hindfoot varus deformity.

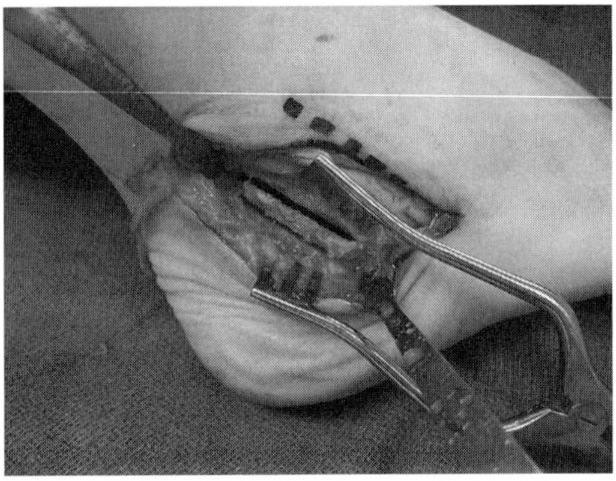

Fig. 26. Biplanar calcaneal osteotomy.

Treatment of associated pathology

In patients with concomitant ankle instability confirmed with stress radiographs, an ankle reconstruction can be performed in the same setting. If the peroneal brevis is split longitudinally, the anterior portion can be used in a modified Chrisman-Snook procedure to reconstruct the lateral ankle ligaments. A posteriorly modified Brostrom-Gould procedure [18] can also be performed in patients who are better served with a lateral ligament repair, such as dancers. In patients with a hindfoot varus deformity, a biplanar wedge calcaneal osteotomy can be performed through the same incision (Figs. 25 and 26). Peroneal tendon dislocation can be treated with a concomitant groove-deepening procedure. Also, a lateral wall ostectomy can be used to treat calcaneal spurs in posttraumatic patients or to treat a hypertrophied tubercle. After removal of the abnormal bone, bone wax is applied.

References

[1] Bonnin M, Tavernier T, Bouysset M. Split lesions of the peroneus brevis tendon in chronic ankle laxity. Am J Sports Med 1997;25:699–703.

[2] Borton DC, Lucas P, Jomha NM, et al. Operative reconstruction after transverse rupture of the tendons of both peroneus longus and brevis. Surgical reconstruction by transfer of the flexor digitorum longus tendon. J Bone Joint Surg 1998;80B:781–4.

[3] DiGiovanni BF, Fraga CJ, Cohen BE, et al. Associated injuries found in chronic lateral ankle instability. Foot Ankle Int 2000;21:809–15.

[4] Eckert WR, David EA Jr. Acute rupture of the peroneal retinaculum. J Bone Joint Surg 1976;58A:670–3.

[5] Redfern D, Myerson M. The management of concomitant tears of the peroneus longus and brevis tendons. Foot Ankle Int 2004;25:695–707.

[6] Sammarco GJ, DiRaimondo CV. Chronic peroneus brevis tendon lesions. Foot Ankle 1989; 9:163–70.

[7] Sobel M, Bohne WHO, Levy ME. Longitudinal attrition of the peroneal brevis tendon in the fibula groove: an anatomic study. Foot Ankle 1990;11:124–8.

[8] Sobel M, Dicarlo EF, Bohne WHO, et al. Longitudinal splitting of the peroneus brevis tendon: an anatomic and histologic study of cadaveric material. Foot Ankle 1991;12:165–70.

[9] Sobel M, Geppert MJ, Olson EJ, et al. The dynamics of peroneus brevis tendon splits: a proposed mechanism, technique of diagnosis, and classification of injury. Foot Ankle 1992;13: 413–22.
[10] Krause JO, Brodsky JW. Peroneal brevis tendon tears: pathophysiology, surgical reconstruction, and clinical results. Foot Ankle Int 1998;19:271–9.
[11] Munk RL, Davis PH. Longitudinal ruptures of the peroneal brevis tendon. J Trauma 1976; 16:803–6.
[12] Arrowsmith SR, Fleming LL, Allman FL. Traumatic dislocations of the peroneal tendons. Am J Sports Med 1983;11:142–6.
[13] Clarke HD, Kitoaka HB, Ehman RL. Peroneal tendon injuries. Foot Ankle Int 1998;19: 279–87.
[14] Abraham E. Stirnaman. Neglected rupture of peroneal tendons causing recurrent sprains of the ankle. J Bone Joint Surg 1979;61A:1247–8.
[15] Geppert MJ, Sobel M, Bohne WHO. Lateral ankle instability as a cause of perior peroneal retinacular laxity: an anatomic and biomechanical study of cadaver feet. Foot Ankle 1993; 14:330–4.
[16] Patterson MJ, Cox WK. Peroneus longus tendon rupture as a cause of chronic lateral ankle pain. Clin Orthop 1999;365:163–6.
[17] Sobel M, Warren RF, Brourman S. Lateral ankle instability associated with dislocation of the peroneal tendons treated by Chrisman-Snook procedure: a case report and literature review. Am J Sports Med 1990;18:539–43.
[18] Sobel M, Geppert MJ. Repair concomitant lateral ankle ligament instability and peroneus brevis splits through a posteriorly modified Brostrom Gould. Foot Ankle 1992;13:224–5.
[19] Larsen E. Longitudinal rupture of the peroneus brevis tendon. J Bone Joint Surg. 1987;69B: 340–1.
[20] Sammarco GJ. Peroneal tendon injuries. Orthop Clin North Am 1994;25:135–45.
[21] Shoda E, Kurosaka M, Yoshiya S, et al. Longitudinal ruptures of the peroneal tendons. A report of a rugby player. Acta Orthop Scand 1991;62:491–2.
[22] Snook GA, Chrisman DO, Wilson TC. Long-term results of the Chrisman-Snook operation for reconstruction of the lateral ligaments of the ankle. J Bone Joint Surg 1985;67A:1–7.
[23] Brandes CB, Smith RW. Characterization of patients with primary longus tendinopathy: a review of twenty-two cases. Foot Ankle Int 2000;21:462–8.
[24] Sammarco GJ. Peroneus longus tendon tears: acute and chronic. Foot Ankle 1995;6:245–53.
[25] DeLuca PA, Banta JV. Pes cavovarus as a late consequence of peroneus longus tendon laceration. J Pediatr Orthop 1985;5:582–3.
[26] Brodsky JW, Harms S, Negrine J, et al. Surgical correlation of MRI characteristics of tendon tears about the ankle. Presented at the AOFAS 11th Annual Summer Meeting, Vail, Colorado, July 20, 1995.
[27] Wind WM, Rohrbacher BJ. Peroneus longus and brevis rupture in a collegiate athlete. Foot Ankle Int 2001;22:140–3.
[28] Bassett FH, Speer KP. Longitudinal rupture of the peroneal tendons. Am J Sports Med 1993;21:354–7.
[29] Bianchi S, Abdelwahab FI, Tegaldo G. Fracture and posterior dislocation of the osperoneum associated with rupture of the peroneus longus tendon. Can Assoc Radiol J 1991; 42:340–4.
[30] Wapner KL, Taras J, Lin SS, et al. Staged peroneus brevis reconstruction with passive hunter rod and secondary flexor hallucis longus tendon as a salvage for chronic peroneus tendon tears: a preliminary report of a new technique. Jeff Ortho J 1993;23:85–92.

ELSEVIER
SAUNDERS

Foot Ankle Clin N Am
12 (2007) 697–708

FOOT AND
ANKLE CLINICS

Index

Note: Page numbers of article titles are in **boldface** type.

1083-7515/07/$ - see front matter
doi:10.1016/S1083-7515(07)00091-5

D

R

S

W

United States Postal Service

Statement of Ownership, Management, and Circulation
(All Periodicals Publications Except Requestor Publications)

1. Publication Title Foot and Ankle Clinics	2. Publication Number 0 1 6 - 3 6 8	3. Filing Date 9/14/07
4. Issue Frequency Mar, Jun, Sep, Dec	5. Number of Issues Published Annually 4	6. Annual Subscription Price $187.00
7. Complete Mailing Address of Known Office of Publication (*Not printer*) (*Street, city, county, state, and ZIP+4*) Elsevier Inc. 360 Park Avenue South New York, NY 10010-1710		Contact Person Stephen Bushing Telephone (Include area code) 215-239-3688

8. Complete Mailing Address of Headquarters or General Business Office of Publisher (*Not printer*)

Elsevier Inc., 360 Park Avenue South, New York, NY 10010-1710

9. Full Names and Complete Mailing Addresses of Publisher, Editor, and Managing Editor (*Do not leave blank*)

Publisher (*Name and complete mailing address*)

John Schrefer , Elsevier, Inc., 1600 John F. Kennedy Blvd. Suite 1800, Philadelphia, PA 19103-2899

Editor (*Name and complete mailing address*)

Deb Dellapena, Elsevier, Inc., 1600 John F. Kennedy Blvd. Suite 1800, Philadelphia, PA 19103-2899

Managing Editor (*Name and complete mailing address*)

Catherine Bewick, Elsevier, Inc., 1600 John F. Kennedy Blvd. Suite 1800, Philadelphia, PA 19103-2899

10. Owner (*Do not leave blank. If the publication is owned by a corporation, give the name and address of the corporation immediately followed by the names and addresses of all stockholders owning or holding 1 percent or more of the total amount of stock. If not owned by a corporation, give the names and addresses of the individual owners. If owned by a partnership or other unincorporated firm, give its name and address as well as those of each individual owner. If the publication is published by a nonprofit organization, give its name and address.*)

Full Name	Complete Mailing Address
Wholly owned subsidiary of	4520 East-West Highway
Reed/Elsevier, US holdings	Bethesda, MD 20814

11. Known Bondholders, Mortgagees, and Other Security Holders Owning or Holding 1 Percent or More of Total Amount of Bonds, Mortgages, or Other Securities. If none, check box → None

Full Name	Complete Mailing Address
N/A	

12. Tax Status (*For completion by nonprofit organizations authorized to mail at nonprofit rates*) (*Check one*)
The purpose, function, and nonprofit status of this organization and the exempt status for federal income tax purposes:
Has Not Changed During Preceding 12 Months
Has Changed During Preceding 12 Months (*Publisher must submit explanation of change with this statement*)

PS Form **3526**, September 2006 (Page 1 of 3 (Instructions Page 3)) PSN 7530-01-000-9931 **PRIVACY NOTICE**: See our Privacy policy in www.usps.com

13. Publication Title: Foot and Ankle Clinics

14. Issue Date for Circulation Data Below: September 2007

15. Extent and Nature of Circulation			Average No. Copies Each Issue During Preceding 12 Months	No. Copies of Single Issue Published Nearest to Filing Date
a. Total Number of Copies (*Net press run*)			1700	1700
b. Paid Circulation (By Mail and Outside the Mail)	(1)	Mailed Outside-County Paid Subscriptions Stated on PS Form 3541. (*Include paid distribution above nominal rate, advertiser's proof copies, and exchange copies*)	952	942
	(2)	Mailed In-County Paid Subscriptions Stated on PS Form 3541 (*Include paid distribution above nominal rate, advertiser's proof copies, and exchange copies*)		
	(3)	Paid Distribution Outside the Mails Including Sales Through Dealers and Carriers, Street Vendors, Counter Sales, and Other Paid Distribution Outside USPS®	163	173
	(4)	Paid Distribution by Other Classes Mailed Through the USPS (e.g. First-Class Mail®)		
c. Total Paid Distribution (*Sum of 15b (1), (2), (3), and (4)*)			1115	1115
d. Free or Nominal Rate Distribution (By Mail and Outside the Mail)	(1)	Free or Nominal Rate Outside-County Copies Included on PS Form 3541	122	111
	(2)	Free or Nominal Rate In-County Copies Included on PS Form 3541		
	(3)	Free or Nominal Rate Copies Mailed at Other Classes Mailed Through the USPS (e.g. First-Class Mail)		
	(4)	Free or Nominal Rate Distribution Outside the Mail (Carriers or other means)		
e. Total Free or Nominal Rate Distribution (Sum of 15d (1), (2), (3) and (4)			122	111
f. Total Distribution (Sum of 15c and 15e)			1237	1226
g. Copies not Distributed (See instructions to publishers #4 (page #3))			463	474
h. Total (Sum of 15f and g)			1700	1700
i. Percent Paid (15c divided by 15f times 100)			90.14%	90.95%

16. Publication of Statement of Ownership

If the publication is a general publication, publication of this statement is required. Will be printed in the **December 2007** issue of this publication. Publication not required

17. Signature and Title of Editor, Publisher, Business Manager, or Owner — Date

Jean Fanucci – Executive Director of Subscription Services — September 14, 2007

I certify that all information furnished on this form is true and complete. I understand that anyone who furnishes false or misleading information on this form or who omits material or information requested on the form may be subject to criminal sanctions (including fines and imprisonment) and/or civil sanctions (including civil penalties).

PS Form **3526**, September 2006 (Page 2 of 3)